Gutsy Travels

Joanna O'Donoghue

Gutsy Travels

*Travelling the World with
My Invisible Friend*

Joanna O'Donoghue

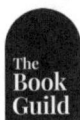

The
Book
Guild

First published in Great Britain in 2025 by
The Book Guild Ltd
Unit E2 Airfield Business Park,
Harrison Road, Market Harborough,
Leicestershire. LE16 7UL
Tel: 0116 2792299
www.bookguild.co.uk
Email: info@bookguild.co.uk
X: @bookguild

The manufacturer's authorised representative in the
EU for product safety is Authorised Rep Compliance Ltd,
71 Lower Baggot Street, Dublin D02 P593 Ireland (www.arccompliance.com)

Typeset in 11pt Minion Pro

Printed and bound in Great Britain by 4edge Limited

ISBN 978 1835741 672

British Library Cataloguing in Publication Data.
A catalogue record for this book is available from the British Library.

*This book is dedicated to my family and friends,
who have supported me through this project.*

*For my children Kelly and Danny and my
grandchildren Ella, Theo and Caspian.*

*A special mention also to Professor Derek Jewell,
who looked after me so well when I was a patient
at John Radcliffe Hospital and dedicated his
life to looking after his patients and researching
Crohn's and colitis.*

Testimonials

A truly inspirational book by Joanna, whose unwaveringly positive attitude shines through each chapter. Absolutely determined not to let Crohn's disease define her life in a negative way, she records her travels to some of the remotest parts of the world, staying in places well off the beaten track. This would be a trial in itself to most people but travelling with Crohn's presents a whole new level of challenge. The lack of access to toilets and the somewhat primitive design of facilities, together with the restrictive diet that is a feature of Crohn's, does not seem to deter Joanna in the slightest.

Doing voluntary work and raising money for Crohn's charities, we learn about her escapades on the Three Peaks challenge in Transylvania, house-building in Cambodia with banana leaves, being on a makeshift saline drip hanging in Madagascar, washing baby elephants in Cambodia and routinely going to bed hungry in Switzerland on her train journey!

The style of the book is pacy, often humorous but always culturally sensitive. I would wholeheartedly recommend this book of distinct little stories as it demonstrates how chronic disease doesn't have to be limiting and can be overcome by courage and determination.

Caroline Hall, Mental Health Practitioner

What a shock when Joanna was diagnosed with Crohn's disease over forty years ago. Gutsy Tales: Travelling with my Invisible Friend *demonstrates her refusal to accept this as a barrier to her desire to visit remote areas of the world.*

The book is a testament to her resilience and adventurous spirit. Joanna has travelled widely, challenging herself with an unwavering determination, often on volunteering expeditions to help others or fundraising for Crohn's, alongside a quest for travel and adventure. Climbing to Machu Picchu and not on the tourist route. Working with children at a day care centre in Quito at a dump. Building a house for a family in Cambodia. These are just a few of the stories she has to tell.

There are some amusing incidents and some quite worrying and even dangerous. Sharing her travel adventures will serve as an inspiration to others, encouraging them to persevere and face new challenges. Gutsy Travels *is well worth a read and I can recommend it wholeheartedly.*

Jane Davies, Retired Teacher and Photographer

Travelling the world is exhilarating but can be challenging at times, particularly for someone who faces the issues that Joanna does with a hidden disability. Her determination not to let this hold her back shines through the book and sometimes we even forget it is a problem until she reminds us. Not only has Joanna been able to help others by her volunteer work and raising money for Crohn's research but she has spread the message about Crohn's disease to numerous fellow travellers and people around the world. This book is an entertaining read describing her experiences in Australia, Southeast Asia, South Africa,

Madagascar, and Central and South America to name a few, which gives readers unfamiliar to these countries an insight into them from her perspective. Hopefully it will encourage others who may face setbacks to push the boundaries and follow in her footsteps. I thoroughly recommend this book.

Jonathan, Norwich

Having read Jo's book of her travels, I was transported to places I could only dream of going to. Jo has shown us how to overcome the challenges she faced travelling with a diagnosis of Crohn's disease. I admire her courage and her honesty. Travelling the world can be an amazing experience. To travel while you have a medical problem would stop most people in their tracks. Jo shows us how to overcome adversity by believing in her ability to know how to navigate the necessary problems. I highly recommend reading this book as it shows us the practical and the funny side to traveling with Crohn's disease.

Rita-Marie Lenton, Celebrant and Author

Acknowledgements

Thanks to my dear friend, Maureen, for her unwavering support to help and encourage me to record my experiences travelling abroad with a disability and also contributing a chapter and encouraging me. I wrote these blogs with the intention of encouraging and inspiring people with disabilities to believe that it is still possible to travel to remote locations, which has inspired her son-in-law, Liam, to contribute, allowing additional insights into travelling abroad with diabetes and a neurodivergent family.

Thanks to the readers who have provided me with feedback and submitted reviews, Caroline, Jane, Rita-Marie and Jonathan.

Thanks to James Homes for the cover illustration (cover design by The Book Guild).

Thanks to all the people I have met along the way on my travels who have been so supportive and understanding.

Thanks to the committee members of the former charity, forCrohn's, who supported my efforts to raise money for research and provided unwavering encouragement.

Thanks to Headway for giving me information about assisted travel.

Thanks to Jerry Bushnell and Tristan Chatburn at DialAFlight for their amazing support with flights and visas.

Finally, to you, the readers. I hope you enjoy my adventures as much as I did!

Contents

Introduction

This is my story. It is personal and specific to me. Not everyone with Crohn's disease would have the same story to tell. Some people will have had much more to deal with than I have and some people much less. But if you are reading this and have Crohn's disease or someone close to you does, some of it will resonate with you, I am sure.

In the early eighties, I was diagnosed with Crohn's disease and it seemed that little was known about the disease then. I have lived with Crohn's for over forty years and in many ways, it has defined me, specifically in terms of the way I look at life. I wish I didn't have it but there are many things worse than this. It has taught me resilience, that is for sure. It has enabled me to learn about myself and it makes me feel lucky for the things I do have in my life. I once referred to it as "my invisible friend". Others would disagree. I am proud of the way in which I have dealt with this disease. It is part of who I am; amongst other things, a terribly difficult dinner guest, but that's another story.

The main reason for writing this book is because I would like to share my story, to help Crohn's sufferers.

I would like to offer hope about the kind of life that can be possible when dealing with a chronic and incurable illness. I wanted to share my passion for travelling and talk about the opportunities and also the struggles which can be involved when travelling with Crohn's disease. I also wanted to describe some of the highlights of my travels to places around the world. Some of the chapters may appear to focus more on these experiences rather than the struggles I encountered, as that could make dismal reading!

I recognise that I have been lucky to be able to fit these adventures around my working life and my family and am fortunate to have been able to save to afford these experiences. I have not included everything I have done, such as two round-the-world trips with my daughter when she finished university and some trips abroad with my son. Two other extended trips to volunteer in Costa Rica and Ecuador could have been included, but maybe they will feature in my next book.

I have included two guest chapters in this book. One has been written by a very good friend, who has recently had a diagnosis which led to her experiencing some challenges with travelling, different from mine but similar in some respects. The other is from her son-in-law, who describes what travelling abroad is like for a family with young neurodivergent children.

I hope you enjoy reading the stories!

Prologue

Getting the Travel Bug

I was brought up in the West Midlands. We weren't rich but we weren't poor. My father was a teacher, and my mother didn't work when we were young. As my father was Welsh, we spent a lot of our holidays in South Wales. I remember the journeys well. I was often travel-sick as my mother smoked and that awful smell of a cigarette being lit in the front of the car stays with me now. She would buy barley sugar and acid drops for the journey to try to stave off the sickness. We would stop en route and my dad would get out his Calor gas contraption and make some tea. We always knew when we were almost at our destination because we could see the slag heap outside my aunt's house in Pen-y-groes, which I always thought of as a black mountain when I was small.

Family holidays were restricted to places in Wales and maybe Eastbourne and Bournemouth for a change. We once ventured as far as Dawlish Warren in Devon and rented a caravan. Package holidays abroad became popular, and I had friends who went to Benidorm and came back with a suntan. There was no budging my father, who had been abroad in the Second World War and wanted none of it!

"Nothing wrong with the UK," he would say.

I found out in recent years that my grandfather in Wales decided to travel when he was seventy-four, having only left Wales on three occasions previously. In June 1949, he left the tiny village of Pen-y-groes with one of his sons to go abroad for the first time in his life. They went on a coach trip to the French and Italian Riviera, travelling 2,406 miles in total. He wrote a journal in beautiful script, outlining the eighty-nine towns and villages he visited. English was not his first language, but I love these sentences on the first page of his journal. He wrote: *My advice to young people is: take a note book with you to note the interesting places you visit. This will be pleasant reading to you in years to come.* I have always kept a journal on my travels. He would be proud of me!

I was allowed on a school trip to Paris when I was fifteen and I remember being more interested in the local French boys than the Palace of Versailles. I reached the age of nineteen without ever having been on an aeroplane, perhaps not unusual back then.

An opportunity presented itself when I was in the second year of training to be a teacher. In fact, that is why I had chosen that particular establishment to train in. I applied to be considered for a place on an exchange programme to the USA and was accepted along with a group of my close friends, including the guest writer in this book. We were to become students at Eastern Michigan University, Ypsilanti which was very close to Detroit. At this time, in the seventies, Detroit had the highest murder rate in the USA and racial riots had plagued the city for some time. It was an exciting prospect, if a little scary.

Taking off from Heathrow, we were all full of excitement at the prospect of the months ahead as American students and the adventures we would have. After half an hour, the pilot announced that we would be returning to Heathrow because we had "lost an engine". That sounded serious but nevertheless was somehow thrilling! Eventually we took off again and the pilot told us that we would receive complimentary drinks all the way. We arrived in New York later than expected and headed off in a big yellow taxi to the apartment we were staying at before we caught the Greyhound bus to Los Angeles. Yes, we went all the way in one go!

I have great memories of this experience as a student and the opportunities it afforded for travel in the USA and Canada, which was so close to Michigan. I took long journeys on Greyhound buses, caught a train to Montreal and skipped off before my exams to Florida for spring break with some American students. We studied sometimes too but not very hard and returned to England six months later. I remember trying to explain why I hadn't completed my exams. The alternative, travelling miles across the country to Florida, had been just too tempting!

This trip did it for me and certainly took me out of my comfort zone. It fostered the desire to travel, to see new places and embrace adventure. I was no longer envious of my friends' package holidays. I resolved to take up any opportunity that came my way. In the words of Jane Austen, "If adventures will not befall a young lady in her own village, she must seek them abroad."

And so I did…

One

My Invisible Friend Appears

1983

Part One: Where It All Began

I am in my twenties, a single parent with a full-time teaching job, and I am living with my two-year-old daughter in a thirty foot-long mobile home. Life is extremely busy and stressful at times, juggling everything. Over a period of time, I seem to be suffering with bouts of cramps and nausea and losing weight. Visits to the doctor are unproductive and I am given various courses of antibiotics which don't seem to work. At one point, I am sent to hospital as a day patient to sit underneath some kind of heat lamp directed towards my stomach. It is not explained to me what this is for, but I have to go every week. I keep vomiting after eating and my stomach seems to be permanently upset, and I spend a lot of time in the toilet. This is worrying and puzzling to say the least. I am also losing a lot of weight.

It is a day in March 1983, and I have been teaching all day and not feeling well. In fact, I haven't eaten anything much, which turns out later to be quite fortunate. I have an appointment with a specialist after school and am hoping for some answers. Somehow, I get through the day. I leave school on time and drive to the hospital. As I enter the room, I begin to sway. Everything feels odd and I collapse onto the floor. I am helped gently onto the examination bed and the doctor asks if he can press my tummy. He pushes and prods and I feel sick. It hurts! The doctor looks serious and says that he can feel a very large lump in my abdomen, which he believes could be a cyst. He tells me that I need to be admitted to hospital immediately. At that I panic, as I don't know who can look after my daughter and, strangely, I am also thinking about the lessons I should be teaching tomorrow. The doctor makes the necessary phone calls to admit me to hospital and tells me to go home to collect a bag and make arrangements for my daughter but that I really need to get to the hospital as quickly as I can. I ask if I can use their phone and contact a very good friend in the village I live in who has a daughter the same age as mine. I try to explain what is happening, but I am feeling very shocked. She leaps into action and tells me to drive home to my caravan and she will meet me there to take me to hospital. She arranges for her husband to pick up my daughter from the childminder. I call my parents in the Midlands, who are shocked but say that they will leave immediately to come to Oxfordshire.

I am admitted quickly, and a nurse asks whether I have eaten anything during the day, as it is likely I will need surgery that night. All I have eaten all day is two smarties and I recall drinking a cup of tea! I am feeling very confused and tearful. My friend stays for a while and the nurse tells me that they need to prepare me for theatre immediately. I am feeling extremely scared.

As the anaesthetic is put into my arm, I close my eyes and drift into oblivion. I wake a few times in the night feeling pain but am given morphine, which makes me sleep. In the morning, I ask the nurses what is going on. I peer under the blankets, and it looks as if I have a caesarean cut. The nurses explain that they can't tell me anything but that the doctors will be doing their rounds soon and will explain everything. When the doctor finally arrives, I am told that I have Crohn's disease, which means absolutely nothing to me. I have never heard of it. He tells me that a large area of my bowel is in "a bit of a mess" and all tied up with an ovary and a fallopian tube, but they have just had to sew me up again as this is a hospital specifically for gynaecological problems. They explain that I will stay here for a couple of days but then I will be referred urgently to John Radcliffe Hospital. In the meantime, I will be prescribed with a high dosage of steroids which will help to reduce the inflammation. The doctor then explains that this is an incurable illness, but I have no real idea what any of this means, either immediately or for the future, and I am too stunned to ask more. All kinds of thoughts are going through my head, but I just want to get home and hold my daughter in my arms. As a committed teacher, I am also wondering what will happen to my pupils, as it looks as if I will be off work for a while.

Time passes in a blur. My parents arrive and friends come to visit. I am signed off work for the next few weeks. I am taking the steroids but every time I eat, I am in acute pain. Three weeks pass. My sister comes to stay. One day, I am in so much pain that I don't know what to do with myself and my sister calls the hospital. They tell her that I need to be admitted. I am examined when I arrive, and the doctor tells me that I need to stay in for a few days while they decide what to do. The next day, they tell me that I will need major surgery immediately to remove the part of the bowel that is extremely damaged, and it is likely that they will also need to remove my ovary, fallopian tube and appendix. I spend the next two days being prepared for surgery and I am told that the likelihood is that I will need an ileostomy. An ileostomy nurse is sent to see me, and she breezily tells me that I can get a bag with flowers on, and it will sit neatly under my jeans. I cry.

The next day I will have my operation, but first my bowel has to be completely emptied and to do this I have a series of enemas. I am feeling frightened at the prospect of such a big operation and even wonder if I will survive it. The nurses are just wonderful, and they hold my hand and reassure me constantly.

Again I feel that needle going into my arm and am told to count. When I come to, I am very woozy. I appear to have tubes coming out of everywhere; there is a drain in my side, tubes up my nose and both of my arms are suspended in the air. I am very groggy, but I ask why my arms are like this and the nurse says something about finding veins for the anaesthetic. I also have an extremely big dressing on my abdomen, but I can't actually bear to look. Later that day, a doctor comes to see me and explains that I have been lucky enough not to have an ileostomy but have been joined up at the site where the large and small bowel meet. I guess that is very good news, but I can't seem to think about that now. I am just grateful to the brilliant surgeon.

I am in a lot of pain and the next few days pass in a morphine haze as I drift in and out of sleep. I am not allowed anything to eat and keep dreaming about food. I tentatively look at my wound as the dressing is checked by the nurses and it seems that I am going to have a scar from under my ribcage down to where the more recent cut is. Many days pass and then it is time for the stitches to be removed. The nurse tells me she is a student nurse, but she will be very gentle. At last I am allowed to go home. I will not be able to drive for three months, and I can't lift anything, even a kettle, it seems. I can't pick up my daughter, but I can give her lots of cuddles. Luckily, she seems to have coped with the separation from me pretty well. My parents go home to the Midlands and a friend comes to stay. We create a little step-type contraption to get my daughter in and out of the bath, so I don't have to lift her. I just have to be patient and let my body recover…

As I recall these events, I wonder how I coped emotionally and, looking back, I really don't know how I did. I know at that point that I didn't want to know too much about the illness at all and rejected the idea of becoming involved with Crohn's and Colitis UK, which was suggested to me. In truth, I think I was in denial, and

I must have been in a state of confusion, but now I know more about trauma, this was certainly a traumatic episode in my life. I don't think I realised then quite how much this illness was going to impact on my life in the years to come. I thought that the operation was going to be the "cure". It wasn't.

Part Two: What Happened Next

I guess what I didn't realise, and no one really told me, is that if you have surgery, it will probably cause more problems further down the line. I was back in hospital by September of that year as I had a "flare-up". I found out quickly that if I ate certain foods, I ended up in the most severe pain imaginable and needed to be admitted to hospital, X-rayed to check for a blockage, put on a drip and given morphine. That has happened to me so many times over the years that I actually cannot remember the number of times I have been admitted to hospital, but without exaggeration, it is probably more than fifty. I began to eliminate certain things from my diet as each flare-up happened. Sometimes it seemed to happen for no reason. This has been one of the most difficult things to deal with, the unpredictability of the flare-ups. There I am, going about my everyday life, when *bang*, it happens. It starts slowly and feels very much like labour pains and this pain increases in intensity until I am climbing the walls and either an ambulance is called (in the old days!) or I get to A and E (also more problematic in recent times).

So began a regime of steroid treatment to begin with. Anyone who has taken steroids for long periods of time will know that they have magical properties but are not great in many ways. I used to develop a "moon face" and put on weight, and they had a bad effect on my mood. However, there were not many options in the early days. Since then, I have been prescribed with a range of medication, all of which I have been intolerant of and had to stop taking. The most recent of these was a biologic medication which I had to stop taking after two months due to its effect on my liver. (Details of this are in my book *Lockdown Stories*.) The most frightening thing about this drug is that it works by suppressing the immune system. This was not a position I wanted to be in at the beginning of the Covid pandemic. Currently, I am only taking a prescription drug which absorbs bile and three-monthly injections of B12, as the part of the bowel which absorbs B12 was removed. It was only after years of suffering with chronic diarrhoea that it was discovered that the missing part of my bowel was the part which absorbs bile. There is a drug which can deal with this, and it has been like a magical solution for me personally.

The other thing to mention about Crohn's is diarrhoea and the urgent need to go to the toilet, sometimes as many as twenty times a day. Imagine your worst bout of food poisoning: gripping pains in your stomach; no control over your bowels; nausea accompanying this; that shaky feeling and then dehydration. Imagine that happening to you over and over again: when you're out and about; in the car on a motorway; driving through a city with nowhere to stop; trying on clothes in a changing room; on a long walk; on a first date; on a bus; on a small boat with no toilet; riding a horse on your own; on an aeroplane with a long queue for the toilet or delivering training to two hundred people at a conference where you are the main speaker. All of these have happened to me and more. The embarrassment of it all. This is something we don't speak about often as there is still stigma attached to talking about the most necessary of our bodily functions.

Due to scar tissue caused by the surgery, I now have a piece of intestine which is referred to as a stricture or narrowing of the bowel. Not only does this mean that there are many foodstuffs I can't eat but it also makes colonoscopies very difficult to perform as the scope can't get through.

Currently, although I had a very recent scare with a raised FIT test result (a screening test for colon cancer), resulting in the need for an urgent colonoscopy, I have had some very promising results which show that inflammation in the bowel is reduced significantly. I am unsure how this has happened but currently my theory is that I have drastically reduced sugar in my diet.

I recently contacted the physician Dr. Derek Jewell, who had cared for me so well all those years ago. He became a professor at the University of Oxford, carrying out research centred predominantly on clinical, genetic and immunological aspects of ulcerative colitis, Crohn's disease and coeliac disease. He remembered me and replied, saying how pleased he was for me that "Crohn's disease and all its misery has clearly been kicked into touch".

Part Three: Living with My Invisible Friend

I have lived with Crohn's disease for so long that it is part of me. I would say I think about it in some form every day of my life.

This is an extract from my first blog, and I hope this sums up where I started from in terms of writing this book. It was published on the forCrohn's website.

LIVING WITH CROHN'S DISEASE,
MY INVISIBLE FRIEND – Travelling with CROHN'S.

That's the dreary part over. Now let's, "Skip to the Good Bit" in the words of the Rizzle Kicks. I made up my mind early on that I was going to fight this illness and not let it define my life in a wholly negative way. I shout about it from the rooftops. I make announcements: "I'm Jo and I've got Crohn's!" When people I don't know try to tell me, "Just try that (food), you might like it" or question why I am in the queue for the disabled toilets, I give them the full facts. People need to know about this illness and how it affects so many people who are sometimes embarrassed to talk about it. I have had fantastically supportive family, friends, and employers. People will urge me to ring them in the middle of the night if I need a lift to hospital and can't get an ambulance quickly enough. They don't even mind if I am sick in their glove compartment, which has happened on the way to A and E. It is hard for them, though, when they see me writhing in agony and throwing up the inside of my stomach lining.

I've had a successful career and have had two wonderful children who are now grown up and I now also have three grandchildren. The second child, my son, seemed something of a miracle as I had half of my reproductive organs removed along with my bowel in that first operation. I imagined my stomach splitting open at the stitch line as my pregnancy progressed. (No keyhole surgery in the eighties.) I have some great scars which I show people indiscriminately!

In recent years I decided to travel the world despite cautionary tales. I have visited Australia, South-East Asia, North, Central and South America and South Africa, to name but a few. I spent two summers volunteering with street children in Costa Rica and Ecuador and I have volunteered in Thailand and Cambodia. I have been in the jungle, the rain forest, up mountains and on remote islands. I have been zip wiring, white water rafting and hang gliding. My fingers are always firmly crossed because if I am not near a hospital I could be in serious trouble, not to mention severe pain. People often ask me how do I do it and aren't I just a little bit scared? Of course I am but that doesn't stop me. I carry a doctor's letter translated into the language of the country I am visiting, some medication and masses of toilet roll and hand sanitizer. Sometimes I have moments of panic but I always tell people I am *travelling with or random people if I need to jump to the front of a toilet queue or stop a bus and go behind a bush. People don't always "get it", particularly the immediacy of the situation when you need the loo but they are usually sympathetic and helpful.*

You're only here once and life is short, so my mantra is to make the most of every moment. Thank you, Crohn's, you may have just made me truly appreciate that fact!!

So, to end this chapter on a high note, read on. In the following chapters, I am going to describe some of the most amazing places I have visited in recent years, despite living with Crohn's. I once bought a hat after white water rafting In Oregon. It said on the front: "Feel the fear… and do it anyway". Let's do just that!

Two

What is Crohn's Disease?

Here is the factual part. I won't dwell on this, as information is widely available about Crohn's disease, but I feel that it is necessary to include at least some information about the illness, although people's experiences of it can vary widely. It is named after Dr Burrill B. Crohn, who first described the condition in 1932, along with colleagues Dr Leon Ginzburg and Dr Gordon D. Oppenheimer.

The Basics of Crohn's Disease:

Crohn's disease is a chronic inflammatory condition of the bowel. It can occur anywhere in the gut, from the mouth to the anus, but the most commonly affected areas are in the small bowel where it joins the large bowel, but it is sometimes present in the rest of the colon. It can also affect the deeper layers of the intestinal wall. One of the effects is that the bowel has trouble absorbing nutrients from what you eat, which can cause difficulties such as the absorption of B12, for example.

It is presently termed an "incurable disease". Patients can suffer flare-ups and relapses but are sometimes in remission for long periods of time. It affects people in different ways. Some people have relatively mild inflammation, and for other people, they require multiple operations, and it affects their everyday life in many ways. Reducing the severity of symptoms and inducing remission are key goals in the treatment of it and this is largely by the use of drugs to minimise the effects or in a preventative capacity.

The exact cause of Crohn's disease is not clear, but it is believed to involve a mixture of genetic, environmental, and immunological factors. Individuals with a family history of IBD may be at a higher risk of developing Crohn's disease. Causes are largely unknown, although research has identified some genetic connections and research is continuing all of the time to identify causes and find new drugs to manage the condition.

Symptoms and Diagnosis

Common Symptoms:

The symptoms of Crohn's disease can vary widely among individuals, and they may range from mild to severe. Common symptoms include: abdominal pain and cramping; chronic diarrhoea; weight loss due to reduced appetite and nutrient absorption; fatigue as the body constantly battles with inflammation; and blood in the stool due to inflammation and ulceration.

Complications:

If left untreated or poorly managed, Crohn's disease can lead to various complications, including: strictures, which are, in effect, narrowing of the intestinal wall, which can lead to potential blockages; fistulas and abscesses.

Diagnosis:

Diagnosing Crohn's disease involves a combination of an examination of a person's medical history, physical examinations, imaging tests, and laboratory studies. Sometimes Crohn's can go undiagnosed for a long time or be confused with other conditions. It is common for a colonoscopy or endoscopy to be carried out to visualise the affected areas and obtain tissue samples for biopsy. MRI scans are also carried out to both diagnose and monitor the disease.

Treatment:

Treatment aims to control inflammation, manage symptoms, and improve the quality of life for individuals with Crohn's disease. Medications such as anti-inflammatory drugs, immunosuppressants, and biologics are commonly prescribed. In some cases, surgery may be necessary to remove damaged portions of the intestine. This can sometimes involve a stoma which can later be reversed.

Living with Crohn's Disease:

Living with Crohn's disease requires a multidisciplinary approach involving healthcare professionals, dietary adjustments, and lifestyle modifications. While there is currently no cure for Crohn's disease, ongoing research continues to explore new treatment options and better understand the condition.

The emotional impact of Crohn's disease cannot be underestimated. To be told that you have an incurable disease with no real understanding or knowledge of how it may progress and affect your life is traumatic. There is support available through patient advocacy groups and counselling, and there is more information available now about the condition than there was. Managing stress, maintaining a healthy diet, and adhering to medical treatment plans can be crucial components of managing Crohn's disease and improving the overall quality of life for those affected.

I would refer you to a book produced and edited by the forCrohn's charity, written by medics, those with Crohn's disease and their relatives. It is called *Book for Crohn's: Written by the Crohn's Community for the Crohn's Community* (6th May 2015) and is an invaluable resource. This book brings together contributions from a wide range of medical professionals and patients. Each chapter begins with a medical professional (including a gastroenterologist, surgeon, dietician, psychologist, IBD nurse) introducing the topic in plain layman's terms and is then followed by real-life, personal accounts written by those with Crohn's. It concludes with tips and suggestions from the professionals and from the patients themselves. Topics covered include: diagnosis; medical treatments; everyday life; diet; surgery; the psychological impact of Crohn's disease; having children when you have Crohn's; having relationships and managing working life. There are also sections written by and for children and young adults with Crohn's disease and a section devoted entirely to the stories of relatives and loved ones. "I think this is just what Crohn's sufferers need. Authoritative, human, engaging and humane, the story is told clearly from every angle" – Robin Phillips, consultant colorectal surgeon specialising in IBD and Clinical Director of St Mark's Hospital. "I have no doubt that this book will become a pocket reference guide to so many people affected by Crohn's disease" – Marian O'Connor, consultant IBD nurse, St Mark's Hospital. All profits raised from the sale of this book are donated to the Crohn's and Colitis UK charity.

Three

Shanghai: My Way

2008

My first visit to China – in fact, the first of many – was in March 2008. I was aware that Norfolk had a partnership with an area in Shanghai called Xuhui, where schools could become linked. I was interested in visiting China and in being involved in this project. At the time, I was an advisor with what was then known as the Norfolk Advisory Service and, amongst other things, I was co-ordinating a project called SEAL (Social and Emotional Aspects of Learning). A local school talked to me about the fact that they were going to visit a school in Xuhui to build a partnership and asked if I would be interested in possibly going along with them. They gave me the name of the person leading on the project, who later became a very good friend of mine, and with whom I visited Shanghai many times in future years. I approached her, along with my colleague, with a proposal for a project to take to a school in Xuhui and join the next visit.

Our proposed project was accepted, and we were told we could go along with the group travelling to Shanghai in March 2008. There followed a flurry of flight-booking, obtaining visas and the necessary vaccinations. In addition, we decided to pilot the project in the Norfolk school where we had first heard about it. The project involved children working collaboratively in groups to plan and design a theme park, using business skills, enterprise skills, and social and emotional skills in the process. The theme park had to meet various criteria, including being eco-friendly and disability-friendly. The children were required to create a three-dimensional model of what they planned. The pilot was successful so we were hopeful that it would be a success in China too, although we were not sure how our idea would be received in the school in Shanghai! We collected a large variety of resources to take with us in our suitcases, which I believe were thoroughly examined when we arrived in China.

Friday, 1st March 2008

We meet the group for the first time at Norwich Airport. There are ten of us, including the Director of Children's Services, headteachers and a deputy headteacher, along with the county representative in charge of the project. My colleague and I feel like the poor relations in this group as everyone else seems very important! We fly to Schiphol in Amsterdam and then on to Pudong Airport, where we catch the Maglev high-speed train, which takes eight minutes to travel 30km and reaches up to 268mph. It takes us to the outskirts of Shanghai where we meet our hosts, who escort us to the Tianping Hotel, where we are to be based for the week.

So, here we are in Shanghai! It is overpowering with so many people, gigantic skyscrapers and the heavy traffic. I had read that the current population of Shanghai was just over twenty-one million. Fighting off jet lag, we are taken for lunch and have to make huge efforts to stay awake until the evening, adapting to the new time zone, as we are told we are to be taken on an escorted trip to see some of the sights of Shanghai tomorrow.

In the morning, I feel refreshed and choose the English breakfast delicacies rather than the Chinese ones. I need to treat my stomach gently to begin with. First, we visit the Yuyuan Gardens with its zigzag bridges, ponds, rockeries and pavilions, then the Oriental Pearl Tower with its glass-bottomed viewing platform, the Jin Mao Tower and the Bund. Again, an exquisite lunch is laid on for us in a tea house near the gardens. Our Chinese hosts could not be more accommodating in welcoming us to their city. They tell us that during the week they will also take us to the Xintiandi area after school one day and on an evening river cruise on the Huangpu River. It is going to be a jam-packed week of new experiences.

On Monday, I wake up wondering how our project is going to go down and I feel a little bit anxious but excited at the same time. My colleague and I meet in the lobby along with the deputy headteacher from the English school and we are driven to the school called Changle in the district of Xuhui. What a welcome! We arrive to see lines of children waving flowers and flags and singing. I have never felt so important in my life! The headteacher meets us and a representative from the Education Bureau and we are presented with large bouquets of flowers as we walk into the school. Massive signs greet us in the hallway: "Warm welcome to our dear friends from Norfolk". We are taken to the staff room where we are showered with gifts. We are introduced to some teachers and a group of children, who tell us all about their school. Many of the teachers, including the headteacher, don't speak English, but there are interpreters on hand and the children are pretty impressive.

Later that day, we attend a meeting about signing up to the partnership. This is the first of several of these more formal meetings with all of the schools in the project. It is very official but several times during this meeting, a mobile would ring, and the owner would dive underneath the table to take the call. The etiquette is quite different here!

The next day, we are to embark on our project with the children. Again, we are met at the hotel and are escorted to the school and taken into a large hall with around fifty excited students and teachers who are going to observe our antics. There is also an interpreter on hand with a microphone who will explain to the children in Chinese what we are asking them to do. Some of the children speak pretty good English, more so than most of the teachers certainly, and they begin to grasp what we are asking them to do quite quickly. They are extremely enthusiastic because they don't generally work in this kind of way as they are used to more structured activities. I can see the teachers looking a bit nervous as they are not used to the children being so noisy. The children are loving it and interacting with great zeal. They are also very good at it and are coming up with some amazing ideas. At the end of the day, we are pretty exhausted but feel that it is going well. That evening, we are taken for a lavish meal, and I am very careful about what I eat. It is difficult to explain my predicament to my hosts and I really don't want to offend.

We are met again in the morning to be taken to Changle to continue with the project. The children burst into the room, eager to continue with the work, and many of them have brought in little gifts for us from home. The day is busy, and the projects come together. At the end of the day, we vote for the winning team and present them with certificates and T-shirts. It has been a resounding success, but I am really not sure what our Chinese partners think about all of this!

On Wednesday, we are invited to participate in all kinds of activities in the school. First, we are asked to put on some white jackets and trousers and are taught some martial arts. Next, I have a game of table tennis with the headteacher. He is very good, and I am not too bad myself, having spent a lot of time in the sixth form common room when I was at school, honing my skills. It's been a while since I have played though. We also do some dancing and some calligraphy. I am asked to deliver a lesson tomorrow which will be observed by the Chinese teachers, and I have a moment of panic. I'll have to think about that later. We are to be taken after school to an area called Xintiandi and later that evening we are to be treated to an evening river cruise on the Huangpu River.

I don't have much time to think of a lesson to deliver tomorrow, as we get back to the hotel late, so I decide that I will do some drama as I can more or less do that off the top of my head. The next morning, I am escorted to a lecture theatre and asked to go ahead. I explain that I need a big open space to carry out this lesson and again I am met with puzzled expressions. We relocate and I embark on my lesson. First of all, I try to say in Chinese, "Good morning and I am very happy to be in your school." The children fall about laughing and the teachers look embarrassed. My Chinese lessons didn't pay off then. We have a lot of fun and once again the children engage in whatever I ask them to do with great enthusiasm. The teachers stand at the side looking serious and talking notes. After the lesson, the children give me more gifts.

I haven't yet mentioned the cold inside the school. It is freezing! It is the middle of March and schools are not heated in the winter. The windows are all wide open all of the time. The teachers all wear their outdoor coats, and the children are dressed in the school uniform of tracksuits. They don't appear to feel the cold, but I certainly do and keep my coat on.

Aside from the cold, I also need to mention the challenges of the toilets and the food for me dealing with Crohn's. The first time I need the toilet, I am given directions, but I seem to go to the wrong place and realise I am in the children's toilets. This consists of a trough down the middle of the room filled with water, no doors, and it seems you need to squat over the top of the trough to use the toilet, apparently in full view of everybody, which seems extremely strange. I am worried that a child might appear, and this doesn't feel right at all. I then discover a staff toilet. I should have asked about this in the first place. The staff toilet is also a hole-in-the-floor type of arrangement and it doesn't smell too great, but it has a lot of candles and reed diffusers to disguise the overpowering smell. I experience a few difficulties. If you have Crohn's disease and you suffer with constant diarrhoea, then squatting over a toilet is really not the easiest thing to do, as you can easily miscalculate. You can imagine the rest.

The food is delicious I am sure but not always great for someone with Crohn's disease and, again, I don't want to appear rude or difficult and I want to accept all their hospitality in the politest way possible. I keep having to explain that I can't eat certain things and if I do, the outcome will be disastrous, and I could risk hospitalisation and be unable to explain my predicament. When travelling abroad, I usually carry a letter translated into the language of the country, explaining my condition and the medication required in an emergency. I hadn't managed to bring a letter this time. Today, I am a bit embarrassed when I am presented with some pizza instead of the school dinner, which they have gone out to get especially for me. Sandwiches are not readily available in China, but we are somewhere near the French Concession area where it must be easier to procure these. I am very grateful for their thoughtfulness.

It has been a week full of diverse and interesting experiences. We are coming towards the end of the week and some of our party fly home. I am staying until Saturday. On the Thursday evening, I am told that tomorrow, as part of International Women's Day, there is to be a celebration at the end of the school day, and I am asked to deliver a presentation about the English education system. A bit out of the blue, but I think to myself, *OK, I'll be able to whip that off tonight in the hotel room.* Then they also ask me if I would be prepared to sing a song in the karaoke competition. That throws me slightly, but I ask to look through their list of songs and I decide to sing "It's Too Late" by Carole King. No idea why, but that was one I think I know best and can possibly sing.

The next day, I arrive at the school, and it is announced that I will be taken to visit a teacher's house for tea and cake this afternoon but first we will have a look around a part of the city I haven't seen before. I am very grateful and off we go. Eventually, we head to the teacher's apartment, where we sit on the sofa drinking tea. The room we sit in also contains her bed. As usual, a photographer has accompanied us. I ask if I can visit the toilet. The photographer accompanies me and for a moment I think he is going to come in with me and take a picture of me on the toilet, but I wave him away politely and he waits for me outside the door.

But the events of the day are not over yet. We head back to the school, and I take to the podium to make my speech, hastily planned last night. I have an interpreter next to me and I begin the speech with everybody in the audience chattering away with lots of sweets in front of them and sweet wrappers being crunched noisily. I could really have been talking about anything, but I persevere and receive enormous applause and another beautiful bouquet of flowers. We then move on to the main event: the karaoke competition. I am called onto the stage to perform my song amongst a lot of very polite clapping. I think someone fixes the score as I seem to do rather well. Suddenly, I am called back on stage again to sing another song with some of the Chinese teachers.

I say, "Oh, I don't think I can do this because I don't know any Chinese songs."

And then I realise that, behind me, the words to "Do Re Mi" from *The Sound of Music* are on the screen. So here I am, a long way from home, singing a karaoke song from *The Sound of Music* with some Chinese teachers in a chilly hall, wearing a long skirt, a velvet jacket, a scarf and some big furry boots. I think to myself that this is a very weird Friday afternoon and an International Women's Day to remember!

Later that night, the remaining members of the English group visit a very unusual German bar, where we drink beer and dance until late. We have to persuade one of the headteachers that we must go back to the hotel for a sleep before catching our flight in the morning, although he seems keen to stay out until the next morning. When in Shanghai…

The following day, I fly back to England and suffer with a bit of jet lag, but my mind is brimming with amazing memories of a brilliant week where I have been treated so well and I know that I will treasure these memories for a long time to come. Little did I know that I will make many more visits to Shanghai in different roles in the next few years, as an advisor delivering training to teachers and involvement in various other big projects.

I was a very lucky member of a small group who went to Expo in 2010 and was escorted in as a VIP to the exhibition to see not only the China Pavilion, where the queues were about eight hours long, but also the UK and other pavilions. In addition to that, in 2012, I took a group of children from a school I was teaching in on an exchange programme with Longyuan Middle School, but that's a whole different story!

Four

South Africa: Encounter with a Lion

2013

I started blogging in about 2012 and wrote a series of blogs about travelling, which developed into blogs about travelling with Crohn's disease.

First blog post ever! Trip to South Africa.

Well... here it is. Everyone else is doing it and I am sure that mine won't be as funny/interesting/erudite as any of the others I read! Got to get to grips with the technology of blog posting first. In a week's time I will be heading to South Africa and this will be my first visit. My Lonely Planet guide is full of useful tips, especially the ones about encounters of the wild kind, such as: if a rhino charges at you and there isn't a convenient tree to climb, stand your ground and face the charge, swerving at the last minute bullfighter style. As for lions, if there is one outside your tent, lie still but if you should encounter one in the bush do not on any account turn and run as you will be mistaken for prey. Stare it out! Walk backwards if you have to and keep your eyes peeled for any more lions that may be watching on your flanks. As for crocodiles… assume the worst. My hunt for a three-pronged round adaptor has proved fruitless in this country. Too dangerous to try to plug anything in apparently. Car-jacking is a worry and I have been told to wear no jewellery and not to take my phone. Aside from all that, it promises to be minus three in the Drakensburg Mountains where we are camping for two nights. The nurse who I saw this morning advised me to pop over to QD and get a onesie. I have OF COURSE got a leopard print one. Now that could confuse the animals when I pop out of my tent to go to the toilet in the night.

I think I got a fair amount of practice with the robbers in South America but I have not before had any close up and personals with wild animals. (not counting the time the deer jumped out in front of me and hit my car on the A146 on the way to Lowestoft)

Anyway… watch this space…

A tale of two lions. Somewhere in Kruger National Park:

Due to rolling blackouts and remote Wi-Fi-free locations, my "travels in South Africa" blog failed to come to fruition. What follows is a condensed version and a memory which will stay with me for some time to come.

In search of the Big Five, we are prised from our sleeping bags in the early morning darkness by the lovely Mike, our guide. With a slight paunch, a balding pate, OCD tendencies and an annoying habit of saying "yis" at the end of every sentence, he is also curiously... sexy. It could be his ability to whip up a three-course meal on the braai in the blink of an eye or his fascination and passion for things with wings and four legs, but he does it for my friend and me. Like a couple of smitten kittens, we jostle for a place up front with the man, sharing his binoculars and hanging onto his every word.

"Did you know that elephants have their sex organs on the bottom of their feet?"

Me: "Really?"

"Yes. If one stands on you, you're f—cked."

I have explained to Mike that I sometimes need the toilet with little notice, and he rolls his eyes and looks unimpressed. We have risen early and are rolling along in the truck with our eyes peeled when I tell him we need to stop. I assure him that I can just go behind a tree, nonchalantly explaining that I am adept at it.

"No," he says in a voice that brooks no argument. "Impossible. Wild animals here. Do you want to get eaten by a lion?"

"Well," I reply. "We haven't seen any yit!"

On this particular morning, my friend has the coveted front seat. Almost blasé now at the sight of impala, elephants, giraffes and a rhinoceros crossing our path, we demand that Mike should provide us with the real deal today.

"Wake me up when the lions come," comes the cry from the back of the truck.

Suddenly they do! Two lions, one of which looks as if he has been transported straight from Narnia, appear as if by magic in front of us. They pad silently ahead of us, and we follow, cameras flashing and videos rolling. Suddenly one turns. The truck stops abruptly.

"Keep your arms in, no photos and keep quiet," Mike barks. He is kidding. I am not even breathing. I wonder if Mike has a gun about his person.

The lion is six inches from my shoulder. He stares into my eyes, and I stare back. He sniffs disdainfully and turns and walks away. We all breathe out.

"Happy days!" A sigh comes from the back. "Now can we have some breakfast?"

That was a moment!

Next instalment will be from Australia. I don't think they have lions.

Five

Australia: A Tale of Three cities. Australia Unplugged.

2013

Diary extracts.

Monday, 30th December 2013. Arriving in Australia.

They say being confined in a metal box in the sky for twenty-eight hours is not good for your health. I know four people who can definitely confirm this: myself, my son and his two friends. They are going to see some cricket and catch up with old friends and I am tagging along with them for the first part and then meeting up with my old school friends and a friend who I met in Cuba. Setting off in good spirits, we have a plan. We think the fact that it is a dry airline may help: keeping hydrated is always a good idea. We bend the rules a bit by buying three bottles of wine – a white, a rose and a red – to help us along. We also take a variety of pills, such as Nytol and Boots' own sleep remedy to help us on our way to the land of Nod. One of our party takes all of them and we don't hear a peep from him for a good while. My son develops an itch and a twitch and can't sleep at all, his friend struggles with his extra-long legs and I can rarely sleep on long flights, preferring to get to grips with a hefty novel. It promises to be a long day's journey into night, in the words of Eugene O'Neill. The concept of night and day disappear. Eventually we land in Melbourne at 6am after what seems like forever and is actually two days in the air.

So here we are in a taxi to Yarraville, preparing to meet our Airbnb host, Av. We decipher the weirdly numbered apartments, climb the stairs of a grubby block and knock on the door. Nothing! It is now 7am. We call Av, who tells us he is on his way and that we can leave our suitcases outside. Dubious but lacking any ability to make sensible decisions, we concur and head into Yarraville in search of breakfast. McDonald's is sadly the only option. Eventually, Av turns up as the temperature in Melbourne rises alarmingly and my friend's head is attracting flies like a custard tart on a pavement. The apartment is not living up to expectations, but we gamely nod as Av explains all and disappears. It appears he no longer lives here but a couple of his mates do. We shower in an extremely dirty bath and put on our beach attire. I wish I could take a photo to show this, but I don't and can only leave this to the imagination. Suffice to say we look pretty ill-equipped and British. My son says we look like the odd bunch.

The next hurdle is actually to find a way of getting into the city of Melbourne, as it is the day after Boxing Day, which is a bank holiday. There seem to be limited transport options. Erratic trains, no buses, and we appear to need something called a myki card. We give up and hail a cab. The apartment described as clean and close to the city centre is certainly not what was promised in the blurb.

The next few hours are a bit of a blur as we all wrestle with jet lag. We walk in the searing heat to the outside of the cricket ground where we watch a gigantic cricketer practise his bowling. We get in another cab to the disappointingly "hip" St Kildare where we paddle in the sea until a mighty wind blows us into a nearby pub, which is showing the cricket on TV. The boys are beginning to realise that tomorrow's long-awaited day of cricket may not pass muster. England are not doing well.

We leave the pub and go in different directions for a while as I need the loo – the usual story! I bump into one of the boys and suddenly we find ourselves apparently leading a group of Sydney supporters into the city, flanked by police. How has this happened? We extricate ourselves from this situation and avoid being arrested. We end up on a free circular tram in Melbourne before calling it a day and deciding to head back to Av's apartment to go to sleep.

Now we look more closely, we realise that the sleeping arrangements are not as described and there are definitely not enough bedrooms, partly due to the lodger situation. There is a bicycle in the lounge next to a camp bed and some weird kind of put-you-up bed. Eventually we all try to lie down somewhere, and I end up in the rather odd position of sharing a double bed with my son. Now, that was OK when he was a toddler, but he is now in his twenties. But we are very tired, so it doesn't seem to matter. I lie down on the bed and drift off for a moment before becoming aware that we are not alone in Av's gaff. The lodger is home, along with his girlfriend, it seems. They appear to have been on a bender since Christmas Day and it looks as if they plan to continue in this vein until at least the New Year. The music is cranked up to crazy proportions, the beers are opened, and the lodger retires to the balcony for a spliff. He asks my son if he would like to join him, and he declines but says that I might. I don't. He has no teeth and a tattoo on his elbow, not that this is particularly relevant, but I am trying to help you to imagine the scene. We explain politely that we have not slept for several days and this is our most pressing need right now.

He agrees to turn the music down a tad but that doesn't last long. Then the howling starts. We wonder whether it is a dog but then realise that it is coming from the lodger's bedroom. A dog outside appears to be joining in, and we groan and put our heads under the pillows. Fortunately, it doesn't last too long, although the dog persists into the early hours.

After a fitful night's sleep, we all agree to leave and by 7am we are packed and out of there, on our way to a hotel in central Melbourne, courtesy of Booking.com. The best laid plans…

Several Days Later. New Year's Eve in Sydney

After an interesting few days in Melbourne, we board an internal flight to Sydney. This is where I plan to peel off from the boys and do my own thing, except that they have generously invited me to a New Year's Eve party. I take a taxi to the next Airbnb. Knock knock. Surprise! No one home! The taxi driver helps by hammering on the door, but the boys are getting restless as the meter is ticking away, so they bundle me back into the cab and we head off to their Aussie mate's house. I think my son may have been a *bit* embarrassed to have his mum along, but the boys are great, giving me a glass of wine, phoning the Airbnb host and even taking me there in a car and carrying my bag. Chivalry is not dead. I am, however, beginning to lose faith in Airbnb.

My host, David, is of a certain age, probably mine. He said he feels a bit befuddled as he thought I was arriving tomorrow. What is it with these Aussies? I know they are laid back and all but really! However, the room more than makes up for the misunderstanding, with a nice big comfortable bed and a balcony all of my own. Can't wait to climb in it, but first of all I take myself to a little Italian bistro for some pasta. They sit me near the toilet as it is the only spare table for one. There is something sad about eating alone but it is amazing how a glass of Sauvignon can lift the spirits.

Today I walk for miles and explore the Darling Harbour. I have been there once before for dinner in August, and it was freezing. Today is a different story as it is unbelievably hot, but I must say that I don't really like it. I prefer the tranquillity of the Chinese Garden and retreat there for a while.

I mooch around in the Paddington area and suddenly notice that everyone appears to be under the age of thirty. Where are the other people? It feels like *Logan's Run*. Not only that, but they are all beautiful. It feels a bit like I imagine Los Angeles to be but without the irritating accent. I eat in a "healthy" burger place, if there is such a thing, and I am impressed to see that this outlet supports the local community by giving donations to youth and women's services. Now I don't feel so bad about eating the burger.

Oh well… It's nearly New Year here and I will be watching the fireworks from a balcony soon. I hope that everyone back home has a fabulous time and would like to wish you all a happy New Year from Sydney.

Wednesday, 8th January 2014

I do love you Australia. I leave the boys in Manly, after crossing from Circular Quay on the ferry and, as ever, being blown away by the sight of the Opera House and the Harbour Bridge. Every time it does it for me and it looks even better this time, sparkling in the sunshine. Manly is busier than I remember, with everyone appearing to get up at well before 6am to indulge in all forms of exercise. I stick to walking but would love to try standing up on a board and paddling around like the locals. I haven't seen anyone doing this in England.

It is great to see my old friends and members of their

family and we spend a lot of time stretching our minds to see who can remember people, places and things that happened decades ago.

Time passes quickly and suddenly I am on a plane to Adelaide. Now, I have never been here before and it is quite different from the other cities. My friend, Lui, who I met in Cuba, meets me at the airport. He takes me straight to see some music in a bar and he spends the next few days showing me around the city and surrounding areas. Being shown around by someone who clearly loves it so much makes it a very special experience. Endless silver beaches, rolling hills, opportunities for wine tasting, weather not *too* hot, what else can you want for?

The next bit of this experience will begin tomorrow when I am visiting Port Augusta, which I understand is not near anything else except the Flinders Range. Lui is off on business to Sydney for a couple of days for work. While I'm up there, I have been advised to pop into the equivalent of an education office to see if they need any teachers. Apparently, they do! Especially for some of those naughty children who jump out of windows and run off. Just up my street.

So... Melbourne... sorry, I have never been your greatest fan.. Sydney... you come second. Adelaide... I'm liking you more and more and can't wait for the next bit of the adventure. Just hoping we don't run out of gas...

Australia Unplugged

I met Lui's cousin, Danny, briefly in Cuba and he visited me in the UK once, where I showed him around our fine city of Norwich, which mainly involved dancing and drinking mojitos in Revolución de Cuba. Now I am in South Australia, Danny is eager to show me his fine city, Port Augusta, aka the Gateway to the North Port, also called "the crossroads of Australia", where the outback meets the ocean. Lui once described Danny as an over-exuberant puppy. Add to that an excessive chain-smoking, beer-drinking habit, along with a liking for some less legal substances, and you get the picture. The more Danny drinks, smokes and "tunes up", the more his eyes disappear somewhere into the back of his head and his smile gets wider until it almost splits his face in two. I am in his hands for the next twenty-four hours or so.

Heading north out of Adelaide, we drive for three hours through the wheat belt. Eventually, the sight of the power station signals our arrival in Port Augusta where roads lead to Sydney (1,500km), Darwin (3,000km), Perth (3,000km) and Alice Springs (1,200km) with not a lot in between except for road! Danny is eager to show me everything! We see "the shacks" where the locals go to fish and party until they drop, the sunset which bathes everything in an orange light and reflects hues of pink and blue over the Flinders Range, and a lot of drunk Australians. This becomes an emerging theme in the town of Port Augusta. Everything is " beautiful" – Danny's favourite word. After a spot of stargazing, we return to

Danny's house where the family who live opposite are partying on the front porch. A world away from Manly and Paddington!

The next morning, we pack up the Ute, pump up the tyres and head north into the Flinders Range. My self-appointed tour guide regales me with tales of absolutely everything about the area and especially about what we should do if we break down. This seems to involve lying under the Ute out of the sun and making moisture from the salt bushes by digging holes and putting polythene over the top with rocks on top. Fortunately, there is no shortage of salt bush or rocks.

"And watch out for the snakes, man. Just stamp on 'em if one comes near ya!" he hollers. He is my very own Crocodile Dundee. I am beginning to feel very under-equipped with my Ray-Bans, vest top, sandals and white trousers.

We stop to get out at Death Rock, where the story goes that local First Nations people once placed their dying kinfolk here to see out their last hours. The sun is blistering. Locals had told me that a temperature of fifty-seven degrees centigrade had once been recorded in Port Augusta. It is nowhere near that, but my skin begins to turn a violent shade of red almost immediately. My bottle of water becomes so hot that I could just drop a tea bag in it and have a cup of tea. In an emergency, my chances of survival lying under the Ute seem remote.

Danny cheerfully smokes, swears and expertly swings the vehicle off-road up and down mountains and through gorges. It is absolutely stunning. Roos pop up from the scrub and emus dive in front of us, zigzagging crazily across the road. We don't see another living person for hours, or a dead one, actually.

Finally, we call it a day and head back to Port Augusta, where Lui is waiting for us in a bar. We collect him and head off to Danny's jewel in the crown: the contraband bar. This has been set up by a group of locals to allow them to drink, smoke and holler to their heart's content. Large motorcycles lean on their stands outside a kind of shack. It is a *From Dusk Till Dawn* Tarantino kind of moment without the flashing lights. The place is packed to the rafters with huge pot-bellied, beer-swilling, chain-smoking Aussie men with beards that ZZ Top would have been proud of. They are called things like Dickhead and Dickhead's Mate, according to the photos on the wall. I can't understand a word anyone is saying except f—k, and they say that a lot. I am seriously reconsidering my idea of teaching in the outback.

"Hey, Pommy Bitch! How are ya going?" shrieks Lovely Linda, the only other woman in the bar. I had met her briefly the night before when she had obviously drunk a lot of beer. She hugs me tightly so I can only assume this is a term of endearment.

We eventually drag Danny away from his slice of heaven and head for the supermarket and the drive-through liquor store. I then have the absolute pleasure of watching two Australians of Italian descent cook up some seafood pasta and, after downing some evil-tasting shots, the evening ends with Danny playing his accordion on the veranda.

As days go, this will be one to remember. Goodbye, Australia. I have had a blast!

Six

Good Morning, Vietnam! Trains and Boats and Planes (and Motorbikes)

2014

I leave Australia and catch a plane via Kuala Lumpa, where delays mean that I arrive in Ho Chi Minh City later than I planned. The air is still stifling at this time of the day, and I am mobbed by taxi drivers all wanting to transport me to my hotel. One asks me for 700,000 dong and I have absolutely no idea whether that is a bargain or not. I think not. I arrive to meet my travelling companion who has flown in from Norwich earlier in the day. She hasn't ventured far without me, and I can see why. The city previously known as Saigon is quite an overwhelming city when you have just arrived from the quiet city of Norwich.

We eat a simple meal that evening at Allez Boo near the hotel and decide to leave the sightseeing until the next morning. I don't know what to say about this city that has not already been said before. Chaotic. Crazy. Smog. Noise. Crossing the road means stepping out into the maelstrom of bikes, taxis and cars without looking. You have to do it. There appear to be no rules, and they apparently avoid you as long as you keep walking. You get the hang of it eventually.

My sense of direction has always been terrible, but I realise I am having more problems than usual in Ho Chi Minh City. Nothing seems to be matching up. It is only when we jump into a taxi and ask to go to the Ho Chi Minh mausoleum that we realise we have a problem. We are using a map of Hanoi. Obviously, we have not done our sightseeing research very thoroughly!

We shop, have a manicure and pedicure, browse in the markets, eat fabulous street food for less than a dollar and buy Ray-Bans in every colour of the rainbow. Seeking some quiet from the bustle of the city, we decide to have a massage. Well, I do. My friend plumps for the safer option of a facial but is offered a bit of an extra by way of a shoulder massage. My masseur whispers in my ear that he is very happy to give me "special attentions" afterwards. I may have just grinned uncomfortably. This is to last ninety minutes, I am told. He pummels, stretches and massages… my back to begin with. All seems fine. Then he straddles me with a knee either side of my back and gets down to some serious business. At one point, he pokes me and gives me a thumbs up sign to ask if everything is all OK, I assume. My face is covered with a wet towel, and I am thinking that this is really not totally OK. He works his way downwards. That's all I can say. I shoot upright and shriek, "Nooooo!" My friend is still having her facial in the next booth, so I ask how she is doing. I tell her that this massage is a bit unusual, and I have had enough but receive no response from her. I find out afterwards that she had on some kind of face mask which made her face feel solid and it had been difficult to speak.

The masseur is still trying his best to persuade me that I am enjoying this. He turns me over and tries to repeat the exercise. I whip the towel from my face and struggle out from underneath him and put my clothes back on. By this time, a gaggle of Australian men have checked in and by the sounds they are making, they appear to be quite up for the whole experience. I hear a shriek from a girl who says she really doesn't think she wants the "whole body" thing. This must be where I went wrong. I haven't even mentioned the upper body experience. I leave that to the imagination.

Many hours later, we stumble into an expat bar by chance and here we meet Wayne, who attaches himself to us. He is from Australia and just does not stop talking. He tells us he has recently married a hugely attractive Vietnamese lady half his age and just sired his first daughter. Prior to that, he tells us he just thought his willy was for pissing through. Eventually, we manage to extract ourselves and decide where we might eat. The choice is mindboggling, but we opt for somewhere on the rooftop of an old building called the Secret Garden, where I sample catfish for the first time. I'm not sure I like it and worry about the possible ramifications of eating something I haven't had before.

The next day we decide to visit the War Remnants Museum. We look at countless photographs of all aspects of the war. All distressing but particularly poignant is the room dedicated to the effects of Agent Orange. This was used by the US military as part of its herbicide warfare programme. As a result of this, millions of Vietnamese people have been affected, including at least 150,000 children born with hideous birth deformities. We see only a few of these people on the streets, as I think they are hidden away in hospitals and homes. It is not known yet how many future generations will continue to be affected. It is a sobering couple of hours.

After this, a little trip out to the Mekong Delta provides a welcome contrast to the bustle of the city. We have a leisurely row on a sampan while drinking coconut juice from a fresh coconut, a little ride on a horse and cart where we don conical hats and head to a honey tea and bee factory for tea, which is a soothing experience. Driving through the roads bordered by endless paddy fields and watching the workers in their conical hats engaged in their back-breaking work is more like the Vietnam I had imagined in my dreams.

A visit to this city wouldn't be complete without a visit to the Chu Chi Tunnels. The tunnels were used by Viet Cong soldiers as hiding spots during combat, as well as serving as communication and supply routes, hospitals, food and weapon caches, and living quarters for numerous North Vietnamese fighters. I marvel at how small they must have been to fit into these tunnels as I try to squeeze myself in to the top of one. Unimaginable to think what life must have been like hiding underground. In all, at least 45,000 Vietnamese men and women are said to have died defending the Cu Chi Tunnels over the course of the

Vietnam War. These have now been preserved and is all part of the memorial to the war.

The trip continues and I ponder that it seems that in the short time I have been in this country so far, I have sampled many different types of transport, and I know there will be more to come. That evening, we join a group and leave the hustle and bustle of Ho Chi Minh City and board an overnight train to Nha Trang, where we share carriages with families squashed into every available space. Some share sleeper bunks, which I think are called "hard sleepers". Some people appear to be sleeping in cupboard spaces and one old lady is even wedged under a sink. They spread out their food, including the evil-smelling durian fruit, which just must taste better than it smells! The toilets are horrible, just holes in the floor which, as the hours pass, become extremely smelly.

Just as I seem to have fallen into sleep, the train lurches to a stop. It is 4.30am and we hurriedly grab our bags and fall out of the train in a sleepy fuddle. We have arrived and the train speeds on to somewhere else. The first thing I notice is how windy it is, and I feel slightly sick from the motion of the train.

Nha Trang proves to be a disappointment, and the beach town is populated by Russian tourists who have flown in straight from Vladivostok to drink cheap vodka and buy copies of designer clothes. In the afternoon, we decide to relax by the pool, and I have my own personal run-in with a drunk Russian who is lying comatose on the sunbed next to mine. He perks up when he sees me and attempts to engage in some conversation. He assumes I am American and seems to hold me personally responsible for the Vietnam War. He becomes fairly aggressive, and I am tempted to push him into the pool but slide in myself instead.

We kill time the next day and eat some seafood for lunch, which is weighed out from a bucket. We decide to get a taxi back to our hotel and I ponder on the fact that there seem to be few traffic collisions. I am thinking just that as we suddenly screech to a halt to avoid the pedestrians caught like rabbits in the headlights in the middle of the road. Crash! The driver behind rear-ends us. Not too much damage fortunately, although of course there are no seatbelts. We climb out and pay the fare and join the driver who inspects the damage at the back of his taxi. Later in the day, I am hit full on by two girls riding a pushbike, so two personal collisions in one day.

We have to catch another overnight train this evening, this time to Da Nang, arriving again very early in the morning. During the Vietnam War, Da Nang was an important military base for the United States, and it is the third-largest city in Vietnam, after Ho Chi Minh City and Hanoi, but we don't linger. From here, we continue our journey by charter bus to Hội An. On our way, we pass the popular beach resort of My Khe, better known as China Beach, an area that during the Vietnam War was popular with the American GIs and was the red-light district. It begins to rain, and I can sense the change in temperature as we head north.

We proceed to Hội An, still arriving fairly early, and walk around the city. First colonised by the Portuguese in the sixteenth century, by the seventeenth and eighteenth centuries, Hội An became one of the busiest international trading posts in Southeast Asia. It is pretty and fun, with beautifully coloured lanterns strung up in the streets and a little quieter than the other places we have visited, with slightly different architecture influenced by the French, Chinese and Japanese. The Japanese Bridge is a highlight! There are lots of places where you can have clothes fitted and made in a matter of hours, which is something we just have to do. We are pushed and pulled and measured and choose some beautiful silk fabrics to be turned into dresses overnight.

That evening, I experience another form of transport: the motorbike! This is not planned but we emerge from a cocktail bar named Before N After only to find two Vietnamese men hoping to give us a ride home. We gamely sling our legs over the bikes and say, "Slowly slowly." No helmets of course, but luckily the streets are quiet at this time of night. It feels like a bit of a Marigold Hotel moment for a second until we reach our destination and our co-riders want more money than we have negotiated, so there is a bit of a stand-off at the end which rather spoils the magic.

Leaving this place behind us the next day, we board a bus which takes us through the scenic mountain Hải Vân Pass with breathtaking views of the coastline. We stop to look at the spectacular view and it feels a bit chilly, and I am glad of my fleece and long elephant pants purchased in the market.

Hue is busy. We get in a tuk-tuk and weave in and out of the traffic screaming with fear and excitement. After this, we take a little trip on the Perfume River which runs through the city. It is apparently called the Perfume River because it flows through many forests of aromatic plants, but I can't smell anything exotic or aromatic. We wave to the women washing their clothes in the river. From there we head to the Imperial Citadel, which was the emperor's residence when Hue was the capital of the Vietnamese Empire.

Another overnight train ride takes us to Hanoi, where we get on a bus for a bone-shaking four-hour drive on bumpy roads and through coal mining towns to Hạ Long Bay, which we are hoping will provide us with a couple of days of much-needed calm. We pull into the area where everyone is congregating to find their boat and I have one of those moments when I urgently need the toilet. I rush off to locate it and luckily not far away I find the ladies', which unfortunately has an enormous queue. Nothing for it but to head for the gents where the queue is not as long. Pushing my way through and not knowing who speaks English, I try to explain my problem, but I think they can tell by my white face that I am in trouble and step politely out of the way. Phew. Catastrophe averted yet again.

I find my friends and we board our boat called the *Pelican*. The staff drop rose petals onto us as we climb the stairs. Although a little misty, the hundreds of limestone islets provide a stunning backdrop. The word Hạ Long translates as "where dragons descend into the sea" and legend claims that these islands were created by a great dragon from the mountains who crashed towards the coast with its tail gouging out valleys and crevasses. It finally plunged into the sea and the area was filled with water, leaving only the pinnacles visible. We board a bamboo raft and row around the lagoon and peer into caves. On the *Pelican*, for some reason we are upgraded to first class, which promises to give us the opportunity to enjoy more good food, a cookery demonstration and dancing on the deck in the moonlight.

After the trip, we endure the bumpy ride back to the city of Hanoi, which is described as "atmospheric, graceful and exotic". We walk through the Old Quarter, which is a riot of colour and sound, and sample some home-brewed beer, crouching on the little stools by the side of the road as the locals do. The whole country at the moment is gearing up towards the celebration of the New Year (Tết). They place mountains of food outside their houses and shops for the spirits. This can happen any time up until New Year itself. They also burn various items and fake money for the spirits. Houses are decorated with clementine trees and peach blossoms in clay pots, which we see balanced precariously on the back of motorbikes as the locals purchase them from the market and take them home to adorn their houses. We learn that there will be great celebrations on that day of Tết when families get together and celebrate the year gone by and welcome in the new one.

The next day, we visit the mausoleum of Ho Chi Minh, where we file past his embalmed body and finally we eat in Seasons of Hanoi, which is reputed to be one of the best restaurants in Hanoi. There is a slight drizzle, and the temperature is much cooler here. I reflect on the journey through the country. It has been a whistle-stop tour and an exhausting one of some 750 miles. It has given me the chance to get a flavour of the country and its people. My guidebook tells me that nine million people live in Ho Chi Minh City and seven million in Hanoi, and I think most of them own a motorbike. The noise and pollution is overwhelming at times, and I have still not entirely got used to dodging the traffic. I have found the Vietnamese people to be a delight; except, that is, for the very few who have tried to rip us off but that always happens and is part of being a tourist, I guess. They have almost all been friendly, helpful and smiling, and nothing is too much trouble. Apparently, their philosophy is to forgive and forget and move forwards to a better future. There are monuments in every town dedicated to people who lost their lives in the war and a harsh reminder of the suffering these people have endured. I like their philosophy of positivity.

So, it's goodbye, mainland Vietnam, and now we are now looking forward to eight days of peace and tranquillity on the island of Phú Quốc, but first of all we will have a few hours of sleep before we get up at 3am to catch the flight.

The island of Phú Quốc, which is in the Gulf of Thailand, lies eleven kilometres off the south coast of Cambodia. It consists of white sandy beaches and dense tropical jungle and is largely underdeveloped, which is likely to change soon with the impending development of an international airport. That said, I am glad we are visiting before that happens. We are staying at the Chen Sea Resort and Spa, located in Ong Lang, which is currently considered to be the most upmarket resort on the island. It has its own private beach, an infinity pool, an open-sided restaurant, a spa and an army of staff on hand to meet your every need. You can even drink champagne in a milk bath if you feel so inclined.

After a couple of days of this unadulterated luxury, I am ready for a spot of action. Should I try to scuba dive or find a man with a motorbike? Or maybe a boat? Possibilities seem limited as the staff positively discourage you from venturing beyond the confines of the resort, hinting that doing so may land you in trouble and urging you to be "prudent". There doesn't seem to be much else on offer anyway. The only people we see on the beach are polite resort staff offering a lemon-scented cold flannel and ice-cold water or, of course, expensive drinks and food.

Then we spot the sign which reads "Thuy House. Restaurant. Water Taxi. Massage". We creep off surreptitiously to investigate and there we meet an extraordinary group of people. First, we meet a friendly Australian woman who has been volunteering in Vietnam. We discover later that she is an artist and a life coach who paints pictures of female nudes and sells pamphlets entitled *Goddess Guides*. She seems to have taken Thuy (pronounced "two-ey") under her wing and is in the process of helping her to acquire a micro loan. Thuy is an islander of an indeterminate age who has set up a small venture right next to the Chen Sea Resort. She is a tiny woman with immense physical strength and resourcefulness. Alone, she has built her "house" from bamboo and palm leaves right on the beach and has set up a restaurant cooking up local ingredients, which she picks up from the market on her motorbike every day. It is quite a trip for her to get there. She had also been cooking on another beach when she met a collection of people wanting to get back to nature for a few days, so she brought them all back to Thuy House. There are two Germans, one who works for the German government in Vietnam on an eco project, a Spanish girl and an Irish guy, who is teaching English in Ho Chi Minh City. There are also two French guys, who are old friends meeting up for a holiday, as one of them lives in Vietnam and the other owns a shop in Barcelona. They are all sleeping on the beach, lighting fires, mending things, sharpening sticks, building pizza ovens and creating a website to help Thuy. A more interesting and nicer bunch of people you could not fail to meet. We are welcomed into the group like old friends and that is how we end up celebrating the Chinese New Year in their company and welcoming in the Year of the Horse.

Around 7pm, a fire is already lit near the shoreline. A table is set out on the beach and candles are lit. Black fish (or they may be called blackened fish) are cooking on the fire and Thuy is creating a number of different vegetable dishes in a wok. We had begun the evening in a much more sedate manner, having been invited to drink cocktails on the terrace at Chen Sea and watch a dragon dance. Now the sound of "*mot, hai, ba… yo*" (one, two, three… cheers) rings out as we down the local vodka. A different kettle of fish altogether. One of the French guys makes a New Year speech in French about the magnificent location and company of friends, and we all settle down by the fire listening to the waves lapping on the shore. We can see fireworks in the distance at Long Beach and a few people stand on the rocks to watch.

At this point, my friend steps into a rock pool and lands waist-deep in water so disappears back to our room. The French man decides it is a good time for a swim, so, not needing much encouragement, I join him in stripping off all of my clothes and swimming out into the warm water and into the night. He is a much better swimmer than me and keeps dragging me into deeper water. It suddenly seems not such a good idea and a hint of panic sets in, so after a while I swim back into shallower water. When we reach the shore, we have completely forgotten where we have put our clothes. Well, I have, but he may have just been pretending. Eventually, he finds me a towel and I locate my clothes and, tucking them under my arm, I scuttle back across the beach, past a bemused security guard, to our room in the Chen Sea Resort. I am locked out. It is 3am. I knock on the door and my friend opens it and screams at the sight of me half naked, with my hair plastered to my head like seaweed. I look like something that has emerged from the deep sea, but my friend generously mentions Daryl Hannah in the film *Mermaid*.

By morning, my sinuses have miraculously cleared, I have lost my precious flip-flops, and my watch has stopped working. Clearly not waterproof. I decide to confine my swimming to the shallower waters in the daylight from now on. A New Year of a different kind to remember and an end to a great trip. One more day to relax before we head back to England to a cold and dreary March.

Seven

When in Boston... Theatre, Canadians and Chocolate

2014

Quote from *Time Travel*: "There are a few prerequisites when considering a trip to Boston. First, don't go in February."

The last time I was in a place where people were complaining about the weather, it was almost hitting forty degrees. Now I am in Boston and the Bostonians all across the city are saying this is the coldest winter *ever!* Since I joined my son, Dan, earlier this week, the temperature has not risen much above minus seven during the day and that is not taking into account the wind chill factor. Once I have donned the thermals, the ordinary clothes, the thick cardigan, the thick socks, furry boots, hat, scarves and gloves, I can barely waddle. After about ten minutes, even your teeth hurt. Then you go into a shop or restaurant or bar and have to take it all off because you are too hot! Enough about the weather though.

Getting here was pretty easy and painless. Crazy that the National Express bus from Norwich to London took nearly as long as the flight from Heathrow to Boston. I arrive on the same day that I have left, have a sleep and then find my way to the hotel where Dan is going to be staying. I may intimate that Dan is a little bit famous because they greet him effusively when he arrives and when we open the door to the hotel room, we find a note to Mr Roberts suggesting we check the contents of the refrigerator where there is a complimentary bottle of wine.

While Dan traverses the city of Boston going to mysterious meetings and looking for possible jazz talent, I waddle around the city in layers of clothes looking for things to do and places to go. Boston is a compact city divided into areas and easy to walk about *when it isn't so cold!* We are staying in the Back Bay Area, which is one of Boston's most exclusive neighbourhoods with public gardens, exclusive shops and the shiny sixty-storey John Hancock Tower, which is the tallest building in New England. The observatory at the top of the tower is now shut for safety reasons following the events of 11th September. However, you can still go up the Prudential Centre Building to the restaurant on fifty-second floor for a magnificent view of the city. Of course, we manage to go up when it is snowing so the view is a bit obscured, but the snow adds a little bit of magic to the experience along with the delicious cocktails.

So, now Dan is on a train to New York, and I check back into the Boston Plaza Hotel by the park. What to do for the next few days is my next challenge. I decide that I would rather like to go whale watching. I find an information kiosk and ask to book on the whale watching trip please. The man looks startled.

"Not till April, ma'am. Too cold. Perhaps you would be interested in a chocolate tour?"

You betcha life I would! Bang goes the dairy-free diet. This sounds amazing so I book on for the next day. Three hours of eating chocolate with a few "surprises" on the way apparently! I book a ticket for an Alan Ayckbourn play so that's tonight and tomorrow sorted… *in the warm!*

Friday evening begins with a marvellous sandwich at a bakery called Flour and then I make my way to Boston Centre for the Arts where Zeitgeist Stage Company are performing Alan Ayckbourn's *Neighbourhood Watch*. The Bostonians are apparently very keen on Ayckbourn and this is their fifth production. It is typically Ayckbourn, with quirky comedy and dark humour, but some of the jokes about the *Daily Mail* are lost on the audience. The acting does not disappoint, although occasionally the actors find it hard to maintain their requisite English accents.

After the performance, I make my way back to the hotel and decide to have a nightcap. Sitting in a bar on my own is a challenge I sometimes avoid but I am not ready to retire to my hotel toom yet. I order a drink and open up my kindle, although it is a bit dark for actually reading. All of a sudden, a very large man looms over me.

"Hey, pretty lady. How can you see to read in this light? Let me buy you a drink."

Now, that sounds like a line straight out of a movie and doesn't happen much in bars in England, so, in my best English voice, I agree. His six gigantic friends join us, and they are spellbound by my accent, which I ham up for good measure. They aren't to know I come from Birmingham. They think I sound like the Queen. My new friend, Chuck, tells me that he has lost all his luggage on the flight but fortunately not his wallet.

"Hell! I've got a thousand dollars to spend this weekend; let's just do it!"

I learn that these boys are here for "the game", which I gather is ice hockey, and they are ready to party. We chat for a while, but I decline to join them for further merriment. Chuck bids me a cheery farewell and one of his friends, of gargantuan proportions, leans over and kisses me on the cheek.

"Hell! Your accent is gorgeous, and you are gorgeous too."

(Note to self: move to USA or Canada, as may have more luck on the dating front.)

Saturday morning finds me at the Olde Trolley Company, joining a motley crew of tourists for the Chocolate Tour. We start off at the Top of the Hub escorted by an enthusiastic English guide who begs us all to be *excited!* She may have eaten too much chocolate already. The delicious mousse-type confection with toffee sauce is easy on the eye and the palette. Next, we head to the Omni Parker House Hotel, whose claim to fame is that they invented the Boston Cream Pie, which we have a large slice of. Other things to note about this place include the fact that Malcolm X worked here as a busboy, Charles Dickens lived here for two years, and JFK proposed to Jackie at

Table 40 in the corner. After this, we go to the Langham Hotel to experience their "all you can eat" chocolate buffet. After three platefuls, I have had enough and am feeling rather sick…

Tonight, I have tickets to see *Shear Madness*, which is one of the longest-running plays in the world. It is set in a unisex hair salon and the landlady in the shop above has been murdered. Apparently, there is a lot of audience participation, as the audience help to solve the crime. I am quite near the front… what can go wrong?

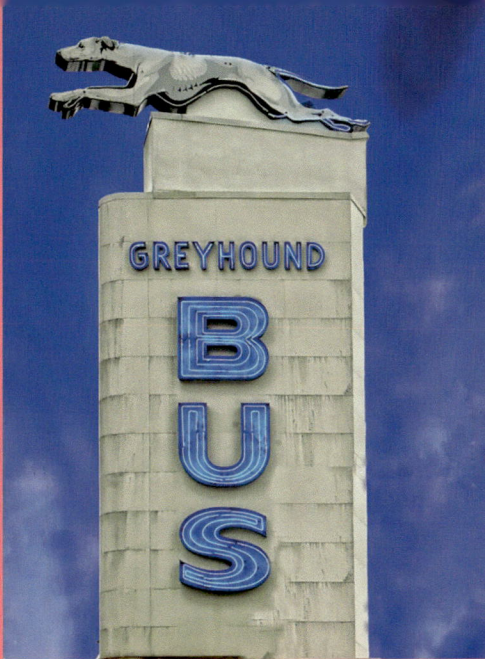

Above: Travelling in the USA as a student.

Below: Living my best life in Thailand.

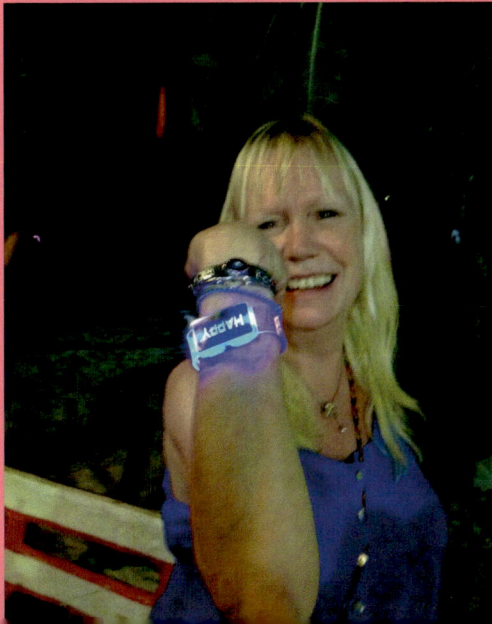

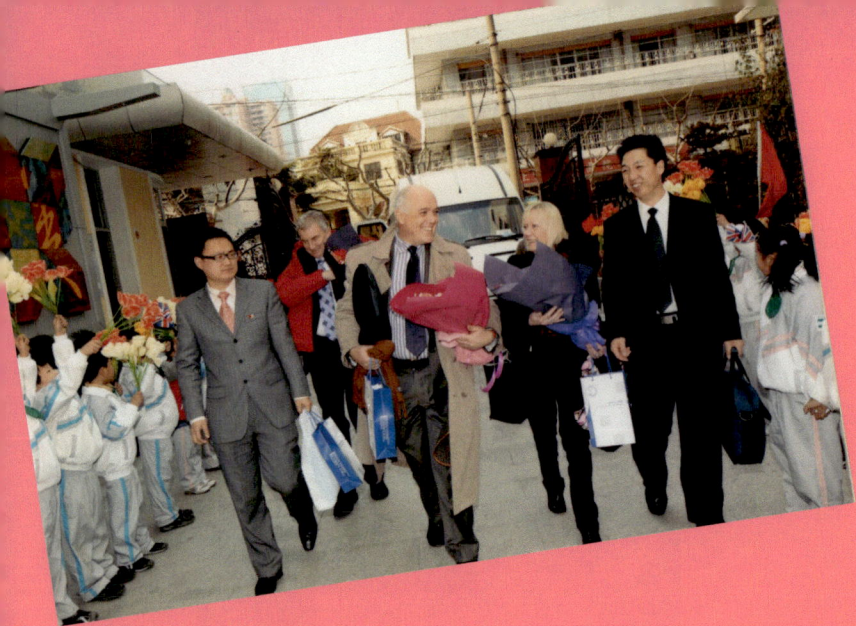

My Way in Shanghai

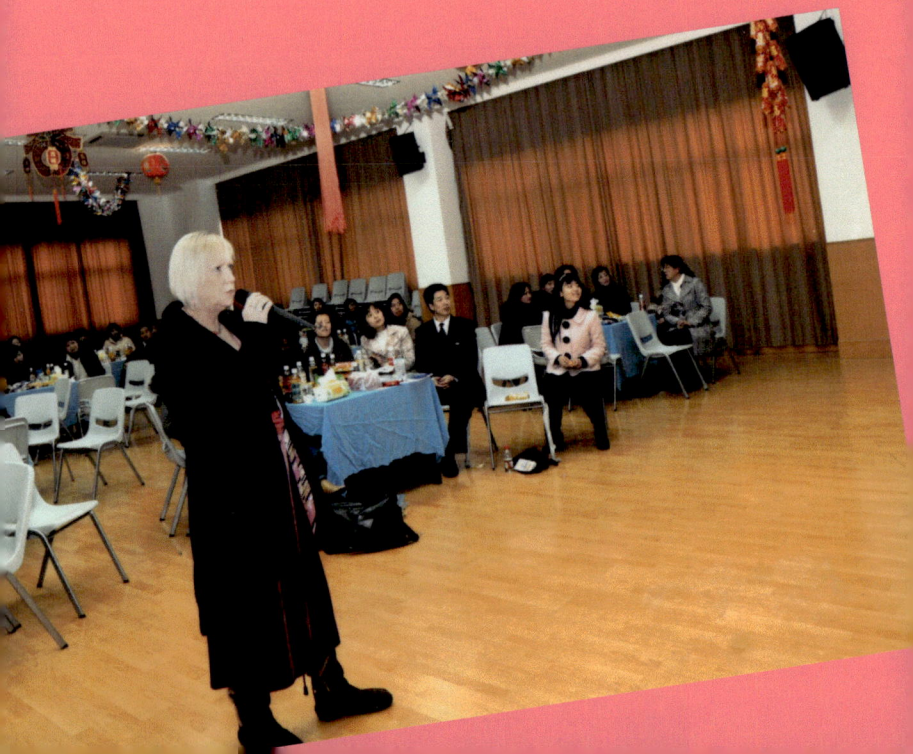

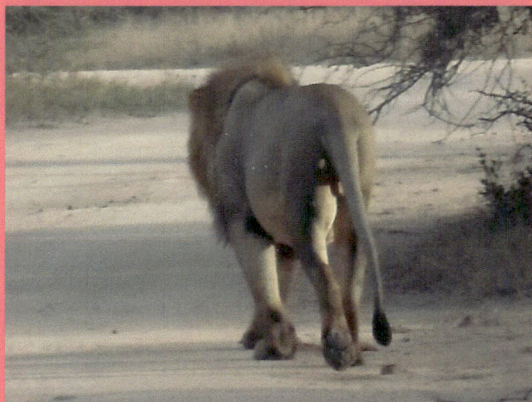

Close encounter
with a lion in South Africa

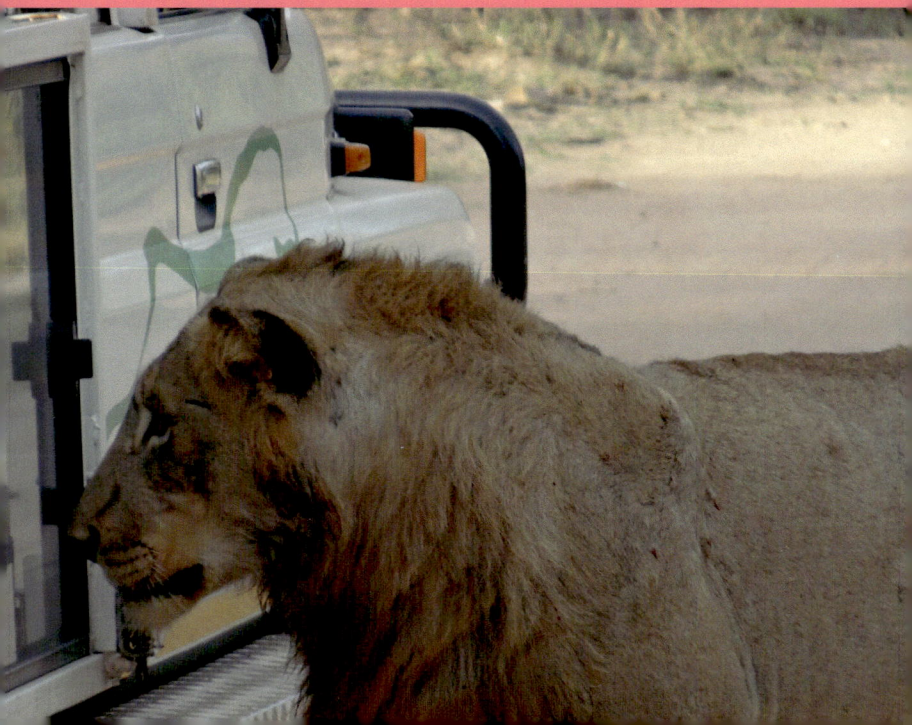

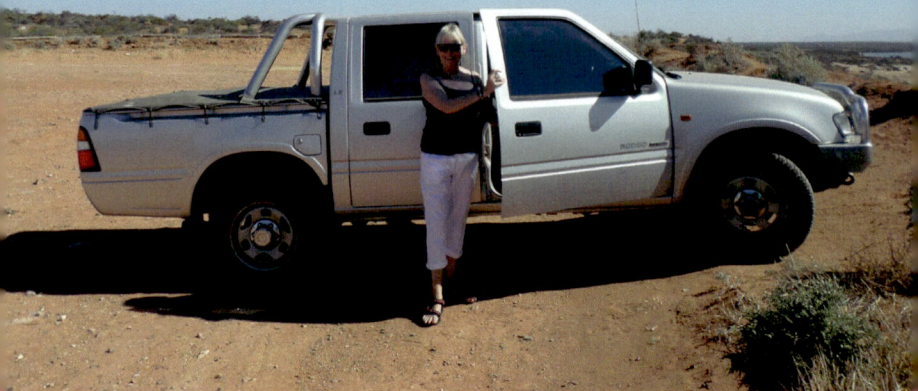

Flinders Range, South Australia

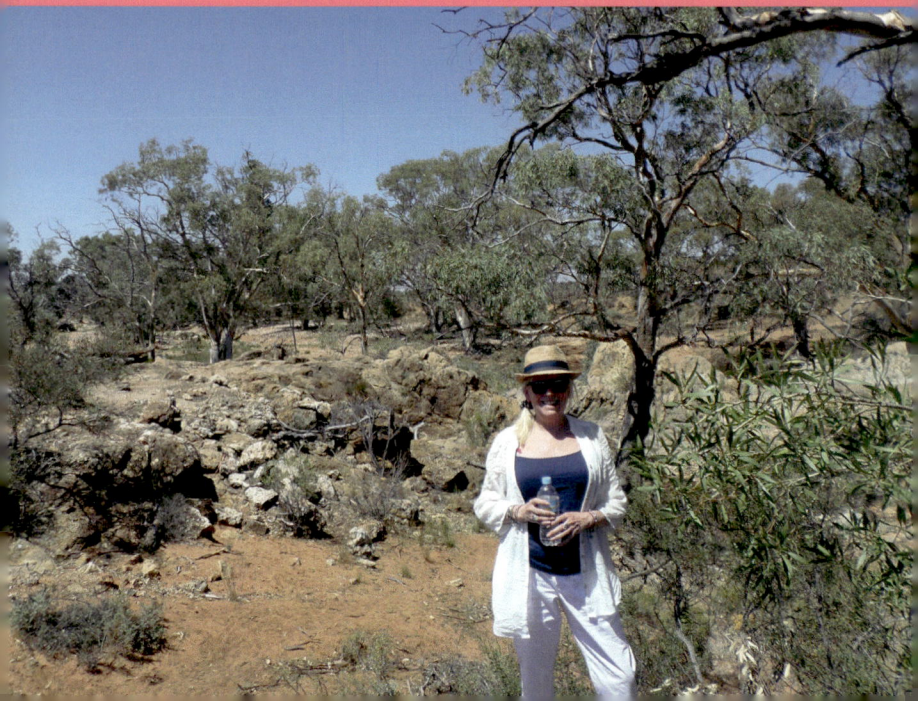

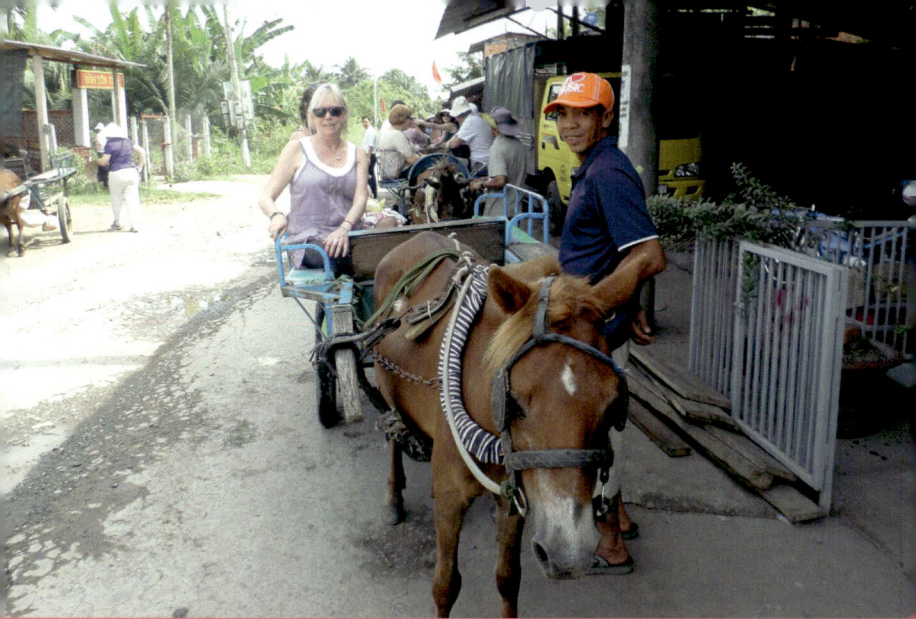

Good morning Vietnam

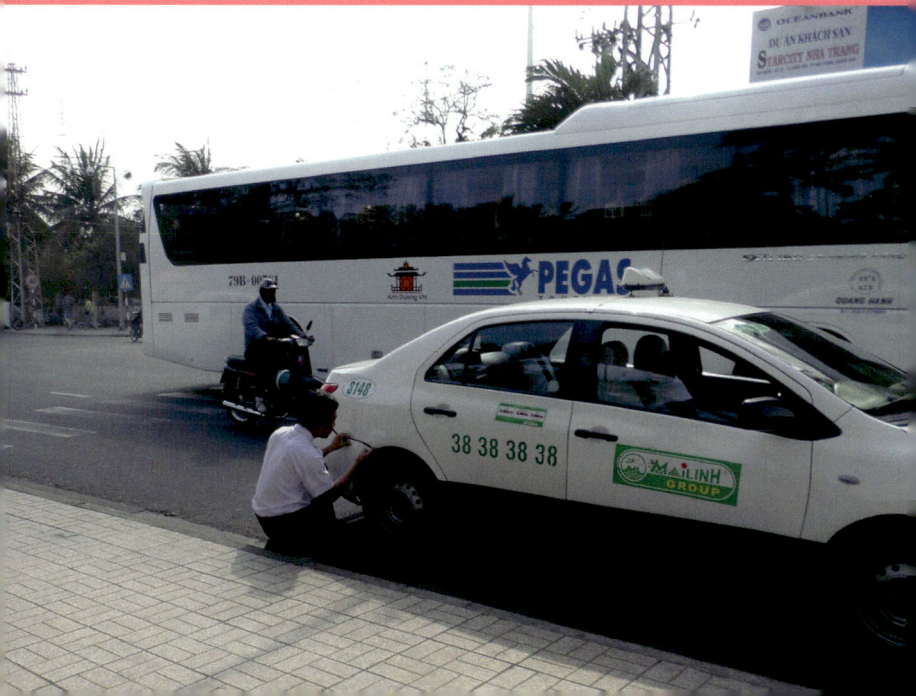

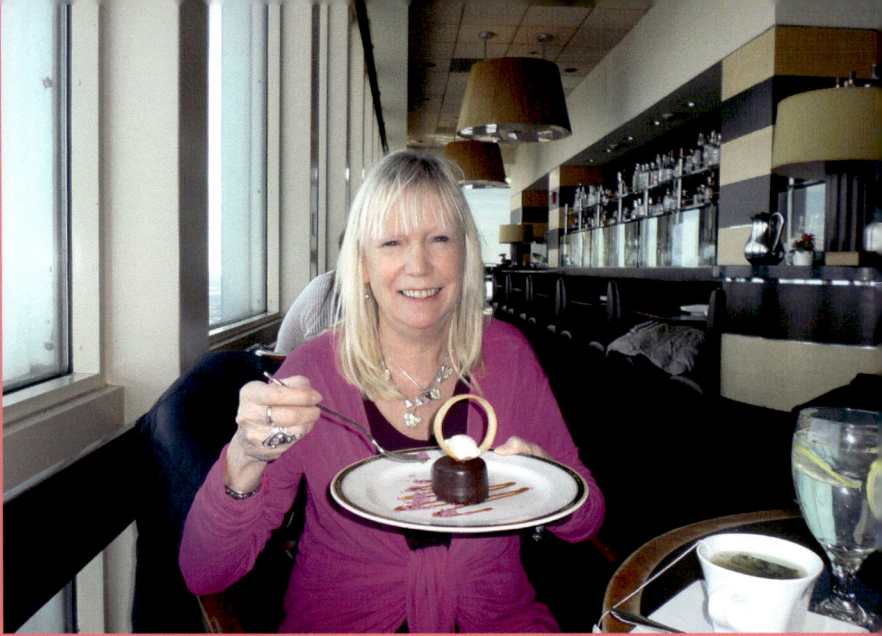

Enjoying Boston – theatre and chocolate!

Plaza Black Box

BOSTON CENTER FOR THE ARTS

NEIGHBOURHOOD WATCH

by Alan Ayckbourn

Old Town Trolley Tours.
One and Only Boston's

Chocolate Tour

Come spend a flavorful afternoon on our most
"full-filling" tour. Visit three of Boston's finest
culinary landmarks and partake
in a sumptuous array of deca-
dent chocolate
desserts from
the city's best
chefs. As the trolley
to each destination, your tour
or shares the history, myths
ds surrounding chocolate as
e watering chocolate trivia

Where

Saturdays Only
January – April

artures

s daily from the
p store (corner of
& Boylston Streets)

cihostly
t the Top of the Hub,
the Langham Hotel's
e treats en route.

ations
ired,
7)269-7010

vailable!

SECTION GA, GEN ADM   BOSTIX EB20228E
GENERAL ADM   15.75   1X
539 TREMONT ST. BOSTON   CN 44973
BOSTON CTR FOR THE ARTS   G.A.
ZEITGEIST STAGE COMPANY   MC210BST
NEIGHBOURHOOD WATCH   GEN
                                    B   15.75
        BLACK BOX THEATRE   ADM
FRI FEB 28, 2014 8:00PM

B50301L SEC E   E4 BOX 1AT   BOSTIX EB50301L
$ 26.00 RESERVED   26.00   5X
$ 9.05
SEC E   74 WARRENTON ST. BOSTON   CN 44232
            CHARLES PLAYHOUSE   SEC E
MC 5X   STAGE 2   MC210BST
ROW E4 SEAT   SHEAR MADNESS   E4

Rock the Kasbah.
Floods in the desert in Morocco

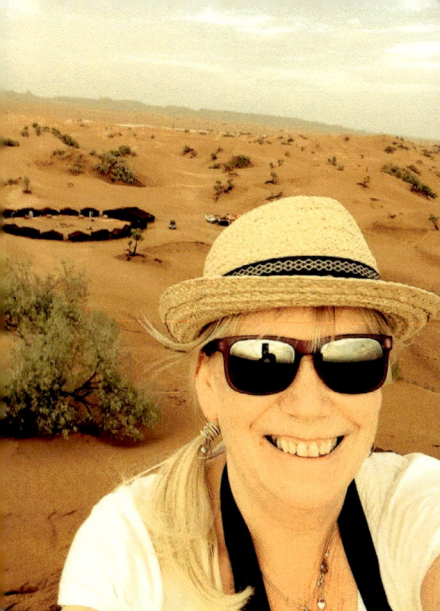

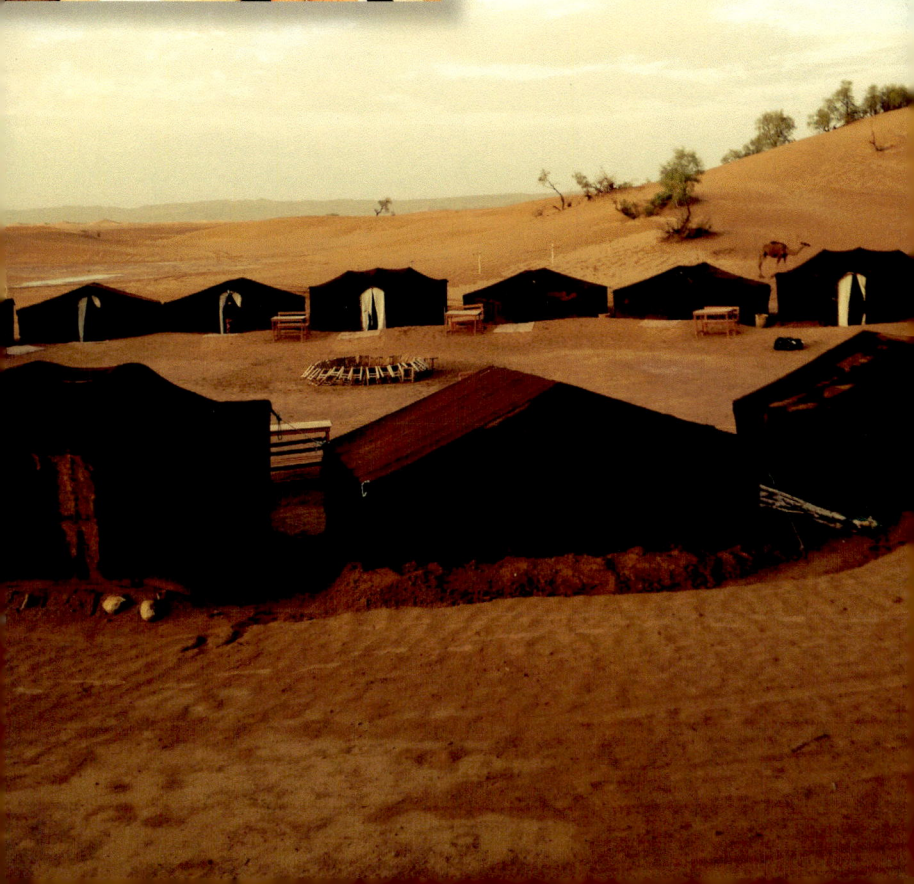

Madagascar.
Tracking lemurs...

A narrow escape and a
coat hanger saves the day

Eight

The Kasbah Trail.
Floods in the Desert.

2014

Several decades ago, I arrived in Marrakech on the infamous Marrakech Express and my memories of the pink city were quite special. On that occasion, I had caught a ferry across to Tangier from Gibraltar with the vague notion of camping somewhere. Not a very sensible idea without a tent but I was about twenty-two and very naïve. Returning to the Moroccan House Hotel in the New Town of Marrakech brings back memories of the previous trip, but I have a feeling this one will be quite different. In the New Town, you could be in any European city, with Starbucks and H&M and a variety of bars and restaurants to choose from. I have no recollection whether this part of the city was even here back in the late seventies.

Heading to the square of Jemaa el-Fnaa, I remember various incidents from the previous trip. Last time, I was chased by someone with a real snake; this time it is a wooden one. This young man is pretty determined to sell me this one and even drops his price from two hundred dirhams to eight, but I really don't want it. I have a lot of miles to cover and don't want a wooden snake taking up space in my bag. I receive my first marriage proposal today, much like the last time I was in this city, although then I was a lot younger! My friend and I find a restaurant in the said square, complete with the ubiquitous fez on the table and a belly dancer to entertain us. I don't remember such things from my previous visit, where my recollections involve donkeys and teeth pulling (not mine) and a lot of snake charmers. Today, although the sounds of pipes and drumming resonate with something deep in my memory, it seems more designed for the modern tourist, with countless orange juice stalls and restaurants lining the square.

Rock The Kasbah!

A couple of days later, my friend and I join the group we are to travel with. We meet to discuss plans for the next day and arrange to leave early to head towards the High Atlas Mountains and the mountain pass of Tizi n'Tichka, the gateway between the great Marrakech plains and the Sahara. Unfortunately, when we wake up in the morning, it is raining extremely heavily. We set off and after about forty minutes, find ourselves in a traffic jam. It takes a while to work out that the bridge we need to travel across has been swept away in the storm the previous night. There seems to be some talk of rebuilding it, so we hang around for a while but in the end decide to take "the long way around". Bubkah, our guide, tells us that this is "a long way" but fails to mention it will take twelve hours to get to our destination for the night. He does not know, of course, that many of the roads and bridges have been flooded and there are many diversions and rock falls to get past on the way. The catch phrase of the day seems to be "it's too dangerous". Hours pass slowly, punctuated by a little excitement when we have to drive through rivers which have once been roads. Bubkah phones ahead and arranges some food and finally we arrive at Quarzazate and are very pleased to stretch our weary bodies, which have been cramped in the minibus all day. We are more than pleased to find a very tasty meal waiting for us. The owner of the restaurant has even manged to paddle to a supermarket and buy us something to drink, which is beyond the call of duty, I think, but most welcome.

The next day, we are up at the crack of dawn heading into the desert to find our camels and a campsite. We transfer into two four-by-four vehicles and head off to find our campsite in the mud. This is not quite what we have been expecting the Sahara Desert to be like. We get stuck a few times in all of the mud and the water, but our drivers get us out eventually. We finally arrive at a little ring of black tents: our campsite! There are a couple of camels on the loose and a Peter O'Toole lookalike who turns out to be our very own cook. We clamber to the top of a sand dune to watch the sunset, singing "Midnight at the Oasis". The view is not as spectacular as we hoped but we are in high spirits, except for my friend, who has been feeling worse and worse in the grip of a nasty virus and a chest infection. The desert is not the best place to be when you are feeling under par. The chef cooks us up some couscous and we toast him with a little bit of our duty-free vodka, which we have been carrying in a water bottle for a few days. It is a bit tepid by now but in the desert, there is not much else to be found.

The bedding is soaked and there are all manner of creatures wriggling about in the sand. I know that I will need to visit the makeshift toilet in the night, so l am glad that I have brought along my head torch, although it makes me look like some kind of mad insect. I suppose this is a challenge for any campers, but Crohn's disease and camping is not ideal for this reason and something I tend to avoid where possible, just because of the inconvenience.

No promise of a hot shower in the morning either, just a jug of cold water to pour over ourselves. The blackness of the night and the sense of quiet is incredible. I have actually slept like a log: such is the unpredictability of Crohn's, so I awake refreshed and ready for the next day's adventure. There has been the promise of a good sunrise around 5.30am in the desert but it seems a bit cloudy today. My poor friend has taken a turn for the worse during the night and a couple of camels are sick, so I give the camel riding a miss and play nursemaid instead. She seems to be hallucinating and whispers that she thought that Lawrence of Arabia visited our tent in the night, or maybe it was a dream? He certainly hadn't and neither had the aforementioned cook, I am sure!

Later that morning, we load up the trucks and head off again into the soggy desert. Deserts don't have roads, as such, but the tracks we are following just keep disappearing into the mud and we almost get well and truly stuck at one point. The sun is pretty hot now and water supplies are scarce. Where are the camels when you need them? My imagination starts playing havoc.

Eventually we join the N12, which looks a bit more like a road in places. We travel through the Jebel Bani, which we are told is a ridge with an elevation of 908 metres but is quite spectacular, and then we head towards the desert oasis of Tata, close to the Algerian border. We stay the night in a dark and tiny room with cold showers and the food is quite unappetising. I am being very careful with my diet on this trip. A good tip when travelling with Crohn's is to take back-up rations if possible so that you don't go hungry. Sometimes I am good at remembering to do this and sometimes I am lazy and forget and then regret it.

The next day, we have another long journey ahead of us, but the scenery of the High Atlas Mountains proves to be breathtaking. We stop at a Berber village and speak to a little old lady who is transfixed by my friend's iPad and is convinced she is carrying around a mirror. She giggles and shows us that she has no teeth at all. We travel on to a place in the middle of nowhere called Oumesnat, where there are clusters of stone houses perched on the rocks. We also see the Painted Rocks, which were created in 1984 by a Belgian artist, Jean Verame, and a team of Moroccan firemen who hosed eighteen tons of predominantly blue paint over the rocks as a tribute to Verame's late wife. We are told that the project took three months to complete.

That evening, our hotel in Tafraoute is a little gem. We catch the last of the sun's rays sitting by the swimming pool and I even take a dip in the chilly water. This is more than compensated for by the fabulous view of the mountains behind. The next day, we decide to skip Agadir, Morocco's top tourist spot and famous for its beach, and head straight for Essaouira, a fortified town with a walled medina on the coast. I haven't visited here before so am interested to see what it is like. I remember that it used to be popular in the late seventies when many people on the hippie trail ended up here. On the long drive, we have to stop several times to photograph goats in trees. We think this is quite cute to begin with, until we drive further on and find some goats are actually tied in the trees, in an artistic way, and there are locals underneath waiting to get money when people take photographs. They are not kind to their animals.

Later that day, we arrive at Essaouira and look around briefly before finding a perfect rooftop bar to watch the sunset and eat freshly caught fish. A well-earned treat after all that bumping around in the desert and the mountains. It has been an interesting trip and very different from my visit to this country all that time ago.

The next day, we take a short drive back to Marrakech into the arms of the Moroccan House Hotel, with its weird four-poster beds adorned with leopard skin, our friendly Cliff Richard lookalike receptionist and our enthusiastic waiters at the next-door Beirut Hotel. There is just time for a last meal together with our travelling companions and to bid farewell to some of them. Nothing left to do except a day's haggling in the markets and a last cup of mint tea. Goodbye, Morocco. I may be back again in the not-too-distant future. I feel as if I still have some more of this country to see and, despite the rain and the mud and other obstacles, I enjoyed it very much and my Crohn's pretty much behaved itself.

Nine

Madagascar: Blobs in Trees and a Coat Hanger Saves the Day

2015

Not really knowing much about Madagascar before the trip, I am not entirely sure what to expect, except that lemurs will feature heavily. Every town seems to begin with the prefix "An" and is often unpronounceable. We fly into Antananarivo, the capital city, which is shortened to "Tana" and means "the city of thousands". Most people know about *Madagascar* the movie, but a lot of people are not really sure where Madagascar is, so for the record, it is off the coast of south-eastern Africa in the Indian Ocean. It is one of the poorest countries in the world.

We see very little of the city as we head east this morning for Andasibe and the Andasibe-Mantadia National Park, where we get our first glimpse of a family of indri, the largest lemurs, high up in the trees. These have black and white markings with a very little tail and a face like a teddy bear, making them look like a panda gone wrong. We spend some time watching a mum with her baby high up in the trees and those with good cameras fight for a place to get the best shots of these. It is not always a good idea to stand with your face upturned to look at these creatures because you often get a crick in the neck and more than you bargained for in your eye. We hear the indri lemurs, who make the most amazing calls to each other in the forest, a kind of eerie wailing sound that carries right through the trees to let each other know where they are and also to warn of danger. We are also lucky enough to see a diademed sifaka, pronounced "sheefahk", which sounds a bit rude. We walk to the nearby village and receive no hassle as tourists but generally are greeted by a cheery "Salama" (hello).

Most of these tours are punctuated by long drives and this is no exception, as we have a lot of ground to cover. We seem to be heading back towards the capital but then turn south on the RN7, which we are told is the only route south. Road is a generous description, as much of it is unmade, winding up and down with lots of potholes, which sometimes makes the journey a little uncomfortable, especially if you are sitting on the wheel arch. This is one of the most important roads in the county and is relatively well maintained in the scheme of things. There is always something new to see on the roadside, either in the form of spectacular scenery or villagers who appear from nowhere every time we stop. It is Sunday today, which appears to be family day, and we pass a river where the women are washing their family's clothes in the murky water, whilst the men cook up great big pots of rice.

We travel further south through the striking scenery which unfolds before us and, leaving the highlands, it begins to get warmer. We learn that this is an incredibly poor country with ninety-three per cent of the population living on less than two dollars a day. Whenever we stop, children appear from nowhere, either trying to sell us something, such as a boiled egg, or asking for a bonbon. They love to have their photo taken and scream with delight when they see themselves on camera. Typically, there are around ten children in each family and families live together in very simple conditions. School is not compulsory and in rural areas children tend not to go to school but work on the land. We see many children working in the fields, helping to build houses and doing whatever they can, including selling things on the road to tourists who pass by. Life expectancy is around sixty years of age and there are not many older people in evidence. The major cause of death is through illness and infections, and medical assistance is hard to come by and expensive.

When we reach Ambositra, we discover we are to stay in a local development which is very simple. Staying here apparently helps this women's co-operative, which is an important base for the development of health projects, agriculture, water supply and the empowerment of women. We stay in a dormitory, share a simple meal and there is no running water and a "long drop toilet". That night, we hear a lot of noise coming from the village. We wonder if there is some kind of party going on. In the morning, we are told that it was in fact a funeral and a celebration ceremony for the dead person. It is known as the "turning of the bones" because after a year, the body is brought out so that the family can say another goodbye and the life of the person is celebrated. Then they return them to the family tomb. They certainly sounded as if they had been celebrating and it hadn't seemed like a sad occasion, but to us it felt strange.

After a simple breakfast, we continue south to Ranomafana National Park. We wind our way through gorges and waterfalls and through rural villages, and we see that many villagers are heading to the weekly market at a place called Robin Camp. We see young men carrying live pigs and chickens and one woman carrying what looks like a flock of geese on her head. Some single men apparently go to the market looking for a wife, so many of the young women are dressed in their "best bib and tucker" as our guide describes them. He has some great phrases!

Our first morning in the National Park involves us climbing up and down through the undergrowth looking for lemurs. We are lucky enough to see many varieties. Continuing south to Fianarantsoa, we stop at a paper workshop to see how they make the most beautiful paper with fresh flowers. We then travel on to the Anja Community Reserve where we see the amazing ring-tailed lemurs at close quarters. We have left the rice fields behind us and now the terrain is becoming dry and dusty. As the sun sets, we drive through the breathtaking sandstone and rocks, the area known as Madagascar's Grand Canyon. We have reached the area of Ranohira on the edge of the Isalo National Park and our hotel is the most luxurious so far, called La Relais de la Reine. This hotel is cleverly built into the rocky landscape and has the most beautiful gardens.

The next day, we wake early and after breakfast we track through the canyons in the blistering heat. We come upon a waterfall and the cold water is very welcome. We see a few more ring-tailed lemurs and then embark on a slightly more challenging walk along the plateau in the heat of the afternoon sun. As we climb down into the canyon, there is a little more shade, which is a relief. I am very hot and sticky and looking forward to a shower back at the hotel. I have spied a place within the hotel for a massage and that seems like a great idea after bumping around for so many days on the roads. I am blissfully unaware that this evening will evolve into something a bit more eventful and will change the course of the rest of the trip for me!

Eating in foreign countries is always a challenge for me. I have been very careful about what I have eaten on this trip so far and haven't touched the extremely chewy zebu meat, which appears on every menu. Tonight, I order tuna fish, as this is always a safe bet and I am tired of omelette. My first bite reveals that it has a very tough kind of texture, but I swallow a piece, almost without thinking. I then swallow a second piece, but this is also strangely chewy, so I abandon the rest of my meal and think no more about it.

At 2am, I wake up with a sense of dread. I can feel those familiar gripping pains coming in waves, which begin slowly and develop over a few hours into a level of pain which can only be relieved by morphine and is usually accompanied by violent sickness leading to dehydration. This is not looking good. This has happened to me so many times over the years that I have lost count of how many hospital admissions I have had. I have sometimes compared it to childbirth in terms of the level of pain and how it gathers momentum but obviously the end result is not the same. I always just know that it isn't going to stop and that the pain will eventually become almost unbearable without the help of strong drugs. I feel a sense of panic engulf me and wait a few minutes to see what happens next. My friend is sleeping peacefully in the bed next to me.

It is no good. I soon realise that I am in serious trouble. I wake my friend and whisper that I think I need a hospital. She knows the drill and wakes up immediately.

"Do you think there is an airport?" I croak? Basically, we know that we are in a country with very poor road links and probably miles from a hospital. It has taken us days to get here from Antananarivo, where we imagine there may possibly be a hospital. The pains are increasing in intensity, and I find it hard to think rationally. My friend goes to wake our guide. She tells me later that she knocked on his door and told him that we needed an aeroplane and that he turned very pale. He wakes the manager of the hotel, and they all appear back in our room. I am being sick by now too. It seems there is no chance of an aeroplane of any description, but a doctor has been summoned.

I writhe and try to breathe my way through the waves of pain. It is two hours before the doctor arrives, as he apparently has come from quite a distance away – I have no idea where and don't care much as long as he can put me out of the pain. He is impeccably dressed in a white shirt with clean cuffs, which somehow seems a comfort as everything in this country appears to be covered with dirt and dust. He is carrying his doctor's bag from which he begins to unpack a variety of things. We are speaking in French, of course, and I am not fluent. He glances around the room and asks for a coat hanger. Puzzled, my friend finds one and after pulling on his plastic gloves, he expertly puts up a saline drip, attaching it to the top of the bed where there is luckily some kind of a rail for a mosquito net. Maybe he has done this before! He plunges a needle into my hand and begins to administer pain-killing and anti-sickness drugs. I keep insisting that I need morphine and not paracetamol, but he ignores me. He turns on his heel and then leaves us to it.

I look at my friend and say tremulously, "What if I need the toilet?"

"There's a bucket," she says. "We'll manage."

The tour guide politely enquires whether I will be OK to leave in a couple of hours? The plan is to drive south and then travel by boat to Anakao on the Indian Ocean. I want to laugh as there is no way I will be leaving this room for some time to come. The manager also looks a little queasy, as I think he thinks I am going to die in his hotel.

He turns to leave, and my friend says, "Oh and while you are here, there is a very large cockroach in our bathroom. Would you mind moving it?"

A few people from the trip tiptoe into my room to say goodbye and then it all goes strangely quiet. The trip departs without us. I am feeling a bit sleepy. My friend goes for a walk and is gone for so long that I begin to worry that she has got lost and I will be stranded here forever until someone realises that I am attached to this bed. Fortunately, she returns and yes, she was lost. She is covered in grass stains. The doctor returns twice more that day to check on me and gives me more pain relief and anti-spasmodic drugs. His final bill totals ninety euros, and I would gladly have paid that more than ten times over. That night, he releases me from the coat hanger contraption and strangely I feel almost better, although a little shaky. When I am in hospital in England, the whole process of recovery takes way longer, and I am usually attached to an IV drip for several days and not allowed to eat. I was impressed with his drugs, that's for sure!

The next day, we stay put in the hotel and I manage to eat a couple of mouthfuls of omelette. We organise a driver who will take us south so that we can meet up with the others and we say goodbye to the manager of the hotel. He deducts thirty per cent from our bill. I think it is because I am still alive and he is relieved to see us leaving. Actually, he is absolutely charming, and it is a very kind gesture on his part.

As we drive south, I reflect on the experience. Has this taught me a lesson? What will my children have to say about this? Should I curtail my travels and restrict myself to places with more accessible medical care? The answer is probably no! The care I have received in this country, which is one of the poorest in the world, has exceeded my wildest dreams. I guess I have been lucky to be in such a comfortable hotel and that a doctor was able to reach me, and I do acknowledge my good fortune in that respect. I feel that someone must be watching over me, and I am not religious in any sense, but I thank my lucky stars that this has turned out so well. My guide and travelling companions now have a lot more knowledge about Crohn's than they did before and that too can only be good!

The rest of the trip proves to be uneventful, and we arrive home in one piece. My daughter's response was good in that she was very casual about the whole thing, saying, "This is something you had always worried about, and it turned out OK." One thing l have learnt is that in the future I will carry a range of drugs and needles with me and I plan to make a doctor's appointment very soon to discuss this!

Ten

Machu Picchu: We Did It forCrohn's

2017

After becoming involved with the charity forCrohn's, I had the idea of raising money and at the same time taking on a personal challenge to prove to myself and others that even with Crohn's disease and everything that goes along with it, anything is possible.

I need to give a bit of background here about this charity. ForCrohn's was a volunteer-run charity, solely dedicated to funding research to help those with Crohn's and contribute to finding a cure in the future. It was run entirely by volunteers, which meant virtually all of the money raised went directly to fund research into Crohn's disease. In addition, everyone on the committee either had Crohn's or had a close family member or friend with the condition, so you wouldn't find a more passionate group of people determined to beat this disease.

The charity was founded in 2003 by two young girls, Tasha and Lisa, whose mothers had Crohn's disease and they wanted to raise awareness about the disease, as there was little understanding or awareness about it at this time. Their first event was a 10km walk around Hyde Park, which was planned as a one-off event but became a yearly event, attracting a lot of participants, and this was the starting point of the charity forCrohn's. It was intended as a short-term project but in the end, over a period of eighteen years, raised in excess of £750,000 for research. A book was also published called *Book forCrohn's*, which I have referred to in Chapter Two. This remains a highly rated Amazon seller and is full of useful information and stories by the Crohn's community. The charity has always been run by volunteers but eventually Tasha and Lisa, both with full-time jobs and young families, coupled with the impact of the Covid pandemic, were led to make the difficult decision to close the charity on 16th November 2020. Remaining funds went to the forCrohn's/GutResearch Grant for research projects. I am proud to have played a very small part in raising money for forCrohn's since I became involved in 2017.

I contacted Charity Challenge and signed up to participate in a charity trek in Peru. The challenge I chose was trekking in the Lares Valley to Machu Picchu and this was described as a "tough" challenge, trekking at high altitude for long days and camping out in pretty cold temperatures. On one of the days, we would have to climb three thousand steps. I hoped to get a few other Crohn's sufferers to come along but despite my persuasive powers, I was unsuccessful in this. However, I was thrilled that my son's girlfriend, Lizzie, decided to come along to support me and raise as much money as possible for the charity.

My consultant was not over the moon at my plans and insisted on (another) colonoscopy to check the position with regard to my Crohn's. Unfortunately, the camera was unable to pass into my small bowel (ouch!) so I didn't know how much inflammation there might be, but I knew that I would have to be really careful with what I ate up there, miles from a hospital. I would have my fingers firmly crossed.

So began the task of raising as much money as we could, with £3,700 being the minimum required to take part in the challenge. We set up our JustGiving pages and friends and family began to donate. We were amazed by their generosity but also that of random strangers, who often had a family member or friend suffering with this illness and wanted to donate. However, we also needed to set up some fundraising events in order to raise as much money as possible. Music events featured in our fundraising, and we held events in Norfolk and at the Troubadour in London, showcasing a wide range of music. We were able to do this due to my son's involvement in the music business and his contacts. All of the musicians performed for no cost. I held two auctions locally, with prizes donated from local businesses, including generous donations from a well-known Norfolk artist and photographer. We held sales in London and Norfolk, a quiz night, and I shook a bucket in Tesco one day. We were able to talk to a wide range of people to raise awareness about Crohn's disease and had some local radio and newspaper coverage to do the same. By the time we left, we had raised almost £9,000.

Alongside the fundraising, of course, I needed to improve my general fitness and stamina for the physical and mental challenges that lay ahead. I spent a lot of time walking with friends and family, joined a gym, walking on the treadmill for hours to build up my stamina and put some strength into my skinny legs! I had a few sessions with a personal trainer and also spent a week in the Peak District a few weeks before the trek so that I could do some hill walking, as Norfolk is so flat and I was going to be climbing mountains.

8th April 2017

The day finally arrives and we meet up with some of our fellow trekkers at Heathrow. There is another member of the group with Crohn's, Ryan, a young man who has been very ill since he was seven. Five months ago, he had a reversal operation and had a colostomy bag fitted again, which will provide him with some challenges on the way, although he generously says they might not be as great as mine!

After three flights via Bogatá and Lima, we arrive in Cusco on Saturday afternoon, where we are to stay for two nights before embarking on the actual trek. We both start to develop headaches. There are eighteen members of the group in total: nine Canadians and nine Brits of varying ages, shapes and sizes. We immediately build up a rapport as we have a common purpose: raising money for our chosen charities and challenging our physical and emotional resilience. Our first challenge is to acclimatise to the altitude, which affects people indiscriminately, regardless of their age or level of fitness. The first afternoon, we take a very slow walk around Cusco, which lies at 3,350 metres above sea level. The next day is warm and sunny, and we have a three-hour acclimatisation walk in the hills above Cusco. At this point, I am feeling confident as it all seems pretty easy so far and my headache from the altitude is only slight. That evening, we receive a briefing from Dougie, our guide, and we are given a bag to pack with essentials for the trip. We are leaving the rest of our luggage behind, and it will be waiting for us when we return. Everyone appears to be feeling bright and optimistic and looking forward to the challenge.

The next day, we get up early and leave at 6.30am, beginning with a bus journey through the Sacred Valley. The scenery is stunning, but the winding road makes us all feel nauseous and leaves us gasping at times as we appear to teeter on the edge of sheer drops into the valley below. We stop off at the market in Lares on the way, where we buy fruit and small gifts for the children we will encounter on the way up in the mountains. We will not be taking the traditional Inca trail but will be following a path little used by tourists. We stop at some hot springs for lunch and then begin our trek, starting with a steep five hundred-metre climb. The sun beats down on us, but we are all in high spirits, although not speaking much as we slowly climb. That afternoon, we have several hours to climb, eventually to four thousand metres and our first campsite at Cuncani. Our guide instructs us to take very small steps and find our own pace and drink lots of water to help to adjust to the altitude and avoid the headaches. I am feeling very confident, but I am really glad that I had undertaken so much training in preparation for this. I feel able to maintain a steady pace without too much effort.

From now on we have a back-up team with cooks, a doctor, two additional guides and arrieros (mule men with their three mules). When we arrive at camp, we are given sweet biscuits and tea to restore our sugar levels and a bowl of warm water to wash in. Our tents have been put up for us and we gather in the food tent for our evening meal before heading to sleep. I have checked out the toilet, which is a makeshift chemical toilet in a nearby small tent. Getting out of our tent in the middle of the night will be interesting!

We compare notes on our headaches, which have begun in earnest now that we are higher. For me, it is a relentless beating in the head, accompanied by a slight feeling of nausea. Some people decide to take Diamox, but I had read that it has some funny side effects, so I resist that.

During the first night in camp, the rain pours down on the tent all night long and it is fairly cold even though I have a decent sleeping bag and am wearing a lot of clothes. I need to make several trips to the toilet in the night and the early morning, which is a nuisance in the pouring rain. The last thing you want to do is get wet and then get into a sleeping bag, but the tent is tiny and too small to start putting on rain garments. We wake early to prepare for the day and climb into our waterproofs before having breakfast and topping up our water as we are advised to carry at least three litres. As we leave the makeshift campsite, we see some of the children who live in the hills who run down to see us. We give them fruit and small toys and they gaze at us solemnly with their large brown eyes and wind-burnt faces, occasionally breaking into a smile or a giggle of delight at what they have been given.

The rain dampens our spirits a bit and we begin with a steep climb. Heads are thumping, we are getting very wet and breathing heavily. One of the girls in the group has experienced a very bad night and has been given some oxygen. Ryan, the other Crohn's sufferer, is also feeling the effects of the altitude quite badly. We climb steadily for two hours with the rain and mist becoming heavier. There is little conversation as people need to conserve their energy. Ryan needs more oxygen and has to rest. There is talk of him being taken down to a lower altitude to recover but after a rest he continues. I find myself drifting to the back and then begin to experience those gripping stomach cramps, which inevitably lead to needing the toilet immediately. I indicate to the guide at the back that I need some privacy and climb (too quickly) up an even steeper incline. After going to the toilet violently, which is not a great experience, I manage to scramble back down but I feel very shaky. We need to catch up with the others, but I begin to stumble and really need time to recover. I decide to do the sensible thing and agree to ride the mule to the top, which is about ten minutes further up.

We overtake the others and the mule scrambles across the rocks to the top. This should be a breathtaking view of Lake Cruscrasa but it is shrouded in mist and freezing cold. My feet have gone numb because I haven't really been moving for ten minutes riding on the mule. A lone peasant woman has seen us coming and sits at the top with her handicrafts spread around her hoping for a sale. I can't believe that she will see many people up here to sell her wares to. We are now at 4,200 metres. After lunch, we climb down slowly for several hours until we reach Wacahuasi, our campsite for the night, which is at 3,850 metres. The majority of us are in good spirits, although several people have had moments of feeling unwell during the day and have become overwhelmed with emotion, leading at times to a few tears being shed. It's hard to explain but everyone is undertaking this challenge for a personal reason.

The next day proves to be the toughest for me. I need the toilet a lot in the morning and feel shaky and exhausted. We are being hurried to get ready to leave the camp, but I feel unable to move from the toilet, even though it is a makeshift one and not very comfortable. I shed a few tears and feel myself begin to panic. What am I doing here? How did I think I could do this? The doctor is instantly on hand to calm me down and he encourages me to eat some porridge with lots of sugar. My head is pounding incessantly, and I do not know how I am going to cope with a nine-hour trek.

We are following a little-used route through the Ranrayoc Valley. We climb and climb and climb. Again, I find myself slipping towards the back with four of the other girls. We slip and swear and breathe heavily, stopping every now and again to regain our breath and give words of encouragement to each other. At the very top, we have reached 4,400 metres and can see the lunch tent way down beneath us. It is freezing cold, and we are being lashed by the wind and rain. As we begin our descent, I feel myself stumbling and swaying as if I am drunk. When I finally reach the tent, Dougie takes my bag pack from me and urges me to drink but inevitably I need the toilet again immediately. When I return, I fall sideways on top of someone, and I am hastily given three cups of water filled with sugar. I am shaking violently due to low blood sugar and the doctor takes my blood pressure, which is normal. After eating some food and restoring my blood sugar levels, I feel ready to face the afternoon. It takes us several hours to descend to where a bus is waiting for us and I have to take several toilet stops on the way, meaning that I am at the back again, which psychologically is not a good place to be. I clamber onto the bus and collapse into my seat.

The bus takes us to the town of Ollantaytambo, where the train leaves to take people to the various starting points to get to Machu Picchu. Our last campsite is just outside the town, and we have a flushing toilet and cold showers. When we arrive, it is dark and we have to organise our tents and some of our belongings, which are to be taken back to Cusco. I start to sneeze and feel my throat constrict. I go to the toilet and look in the mirror (a rare thing to have at a campsite but this final one has a few more facilities!) to see that my face and eyes are swollen, and it looks as if I am having an allergic reaction to something, although I am later told that this could be due to the altitude. I take a couple of puffs on my inhaler and at 7pm decide to call it a day, crawling into my sleeping bag, deciding to miss dinner in favour of getting some sleep. We have to get up at 4am the next morning to be ready to get to the train station to catch the train for the final push to our destination.

In the morning after some sleep, I feel a little better. We eat breakfast and head for the train in the dark. We disembark from the train at gate 106, from where we will climb to Wiñayhuayha and then up to Machu Picchu. The heavy rain has rendered gate 104, with the promised three thousand steps, impassable. We are not to be disappointed, however, as we still have several hours of climbing to do. We start to climb. I don't know why but I have a feeling that this is going to be my best day with the end in sight. We have dropped in altitude, so the headache has gone, and I feel that this is what I have trained so hard for. I keep up with the others, although obviously not the super fit teenagers. Lizzie and Ryan are ahead of me, and I occasionally catch up with them and someone comments that I am "flying" today. We stop for a brief sandwich lunch and again to look at the ruins of Wiñayhuayha and then we are ready for the final climb upwards towards the Sun Gate.

By the time we reach the top, we have apparently climbed 109 floors and taken 6,316 steps according to someone's gadget! A few very steep steps lead us up through the Sun Gate and our first glimpse of Machu

Picchu. It is shrouded in mist and every bit as inspiring and magical as people describe. The sun comes out for us as we stand at the top and just gaze down at the site. As a group, we have achieved our goal, even though some of us have had a harder time of it than others. We take some time to catch our breath and take photos and then begin a steady climb down. It feels odd being amongst so many people after seeing no one for days except for the local peasant communities.

As we near the site, it begins to rain heavily but we are all elated at our achievement. We take a group photo before heading towards a bus stop to catch a bus down to Aguas Calientes, where we are staying for one night. We queue for over an hour in the unforgiving, pouring rain and then endure another butt-clenching bus ride, careering around hairpin bends until we reach the town. We are soaked through to our underwear and have to dry our clothes with a hairdryer, but, bliss, we have a hot shower and a flushing toilet. We head out for some food into the buzzing little town full of people on their way to or back from the site of Machu Picchu.

The next day, we have an opportunity to explore "the Lost City of the Incas" at a slightly more leisurely pace in our tourist clothes, thankful not to have to wear our heavy walking boots and stinky socks any longer. In the afternoon, we catch the train back to Ollantaytambo and then a bus onwards to Cusco where we are to have a final celebratory meal and say our goodbyes to the group as some head home, although Lizzie and I are heading on to Bolivia.

This was described as a tough trek and indeed it lived up to its description, for me anyway. The altitude and weather conditions made it more difficult than I had anticipated. I felt an overwhelming sense of exhaustion at times, but this culminated in a real high at the end, having achieved a personal challenge and raised a lot of money for forCrohn's. The slogan on our T-shirts proclaimed, "We did it for Crohn's", but I also "did it with Crohn's".

We had decided to extend out trip, so the next morning, Lizzie and I say goodbye to our fellow climbers and head for a local bus which is going to take us to Puno. The journey is to take us just over seven hours. I'm not feeling well and on a couple of occasions I have to ask the bus driver when we will stop so that I can go to the toilet, as there isn't one on the bus. On one occasion, I have to insist on him stopping at the side of the road before we reach the next town. It is not usual to do this, but he can see my desperation and the fact that I repeat "*es necesario*" very loudly and firmly. My Crohn's symptoms seem to be worsening. We sleep most of the way as we are exhausted.

We arrive in Puno and have an overnight stay in a hotel. We are met at the hotel by a guide who says that he will take us to Lake Titicaca tomorrow. My guidebook tells me that Lake Titicaca is the largest freshwater lake in South America and also the highest of the world's large lakes. It is one of less than twenty ancient lakes on earth and is thought to be three million years old. Lake Titicaca sits 3,810 metres above sea level and is situated between Peru to the west and Bolivia to the east. It seems that we are still in Peru and not in Bolivia as we thought. I was convinced that the extension trip notes had promised to take us to Bolivia. I don't think I realised how large Lake Titicaca actually is.

We get up early and head down to get a boat, which seems as if it is going to be steered by a ten-year-old boy. He expertly moves the boat so that we can hop on it. We go to the Floating Islands, which are man-made and very colourful. Apparently, these are constructed by the people of Uros from layers of totora, a thick buoyant grass that grows abundantly in the shallow areas of the lake. The people continuously add layers of these sedges to the surfaces. They are golden in colour but are painted in a variety of bright colours. Each island is decorated differently and uniquely from the other and inhabited by individual families who also build different types of thatched houses for themselves on each island. Families in their traditional outfits come to greet us and invite us into their homes, and we feel as if we should buy something, so I buy a beautifully hand-embroidered piece of material, which will find a place in my house somewhere!

We then head on to the island of Amantaní, which we are told by our guide is one of the least-visited islands with a local population of around four thousand people, which comprises eight hundred families. This island offers overnight stays, and this is what we are going to do. Our guide seems vague, and I tell him I will be needing the toilet soon. It doesn't look as if he has organised a homestay, but we are not really sure of the system. Finally, he takes us to a family who seem friendly and keen to have us, so we agree to stay. They speak Quechua, an indigenous language that originated in central Peru and then spread to other countries of the Andes. This makes it difficult to communicate but the older man in the family speaks a little English.

We are shown to a room outside their dwelling and up some stairs, which has been furnished very basically and includes twin beds with highly decorated bedspreads. Down the stairs outside the family's living quarters is a shed which has "toilet" written on it. This is a very basic toilet with no flush and a bucket of water next to it. I have a feeling that I am going to be visiting this a lot! We try to chat with the family, and they are very hospitable and invite us in to have some soup. It becomes obvious that they were not expecting us, and I try to explain my dietary limitations. There seem to be a lot of very small potatoes that they are going to make into something for later and I have to explain that I will need these to be peeled.

We go for a walk and decide to head for the highest point of the island to see the sunset. We are both pretty exhausted after our trek but begin the slog uphill. Suddenly, a local islander goes past us on a horse, and I shout to him. Somehow, by gesticulation and a bit of role play, I explain that I would like to ride his horse to the top and offer him ten dollars. He agrees and I leap on, leaving poor Lizzie to trail in my wake. When I get to the top, I dismount and offer him my ten dollar note but he is very cross that it is not a new one and that is tricky as I don't have anything else with me. Lizzie arrives at the top and we watch the sunset then realise that we need to find our way back down to where we are staying quickly as it is getting darker and darker. Thank goodness for phones with torches.

We eat our potato stew and sit with the family for a while until we feel we can retire for the night. That night is not a comfortable one with the many trips I have to make to the toilet. In the morning, we have some kind of pancake with the family and then head for a boat which is to take us back to Puno. This is not a great ride either as we are told we are not allowed to use the makeshift toilet. We sit on the top of the boat and just hope that we won't take too long to reach the shore. We finally arrive back and head to the hotel and I have to say I don't feel great, and we are due to fly home in the morning. I sway and stumble in the foyer of the hotel and someone grabs my arm and tells me to sit down while they get some oxygen. I explain that I am not suffering with altitude sickness but have Crohn's disease. My body is feeling battered from the exhausting trek and the number of times I have had to go to the toilet, which is more than usual.

It is a long flight home, but we doze. Lizzie has very sunburnt legs due to sitting on the top of the boat in the strong sun so is not very comfortable. When we reach Heathrow we exit with our rucksacks, somehow expecting to find a posse of people clapping to herald our arrival back into the UK and congratulate us. There is no one. Emotion overwhelms me and I cry.

It is only when I get home that I find out that several people from the trek have been taken ill and two of them are in hospital. I go to the doctor and explain my symptoms and he takes a sample. A day later, I find out that I have a *Campylobacter* infection, which I understand can happen due to eating raw or undercooked poultry or eating something that has touched it, or it can be by contact with animals or drinking untreated water. I guess any of those things could have happened during our trek. Antibiotics will sort it, but I am lucky compared with one or two of the others who are really still quite poorly. I guess that is just one of the hazards of such an experience, but I survived to tell the tale, proved that such a challenge is possible, and raised a lot of money into the bargain!

Eleven

Thailand and Cambodia: Washing Elephants and Building Houses

2017

Following my trek to Peru to raise money for the forCrohn's charity, I felt as if I was a bit exhausted with fundraising and continuing to ask people to support me, so I turned my thoughts to planning another adventure. I still wanted to prove that it is possible to travel to remoter parts of the world and cope with the challenges it presents for us Crohn's sufferers.

I found a company and decided to take the plunge and signed up for a volunteer programme in Thailand and Cambodia. All I knew was that the company was based in New Zealand and this particular trip was called "Young at Heart". I hate that expression. It was described like this: "This most popular volunteer tour takes you through two of Southeast Asia's most exciting countries with a group of like-minded people, fully supported by experienced guides". This was more of their blurb: "It is the next step in independent volunteering and adventure travel. We're dedicated to pushing the boundaries of what responsible tourism is all about. Our dedicated team, consisting of the perfect mix of international travellers and passionate locals, know exactly how to ensure that both you, our hearty traveller, and the communities that we're dedicated to support, receive the very best adventure, fun, financial help, support, care, love, hugs and hi-5's! Where we go, we leave footprints.

"Starting in Thailand's iconic capital, Bangkok, you'll travel to the north-eastern province of Surin for an unforgettable few days getting up close and personal with the majestic elephants and living amongst the beautiful people that call this place home. Help out with micro development projects which benefit not only the welfare of the elephants but also the local communities that protect them. After five days here, waving goodbye to your new-found friends you'll head over the border to Cambodia and on to the chilled-out city of Siem Reap. Here you'll get to work with NGOs at various community projects as well as experience the awesome temples of Angkor Wat."

I had previously engaged in a couple of projects for volunteers in Central and South America and had some reservations about companies which claim all sorts of things but are actually just a money-making enterprise (more of this at the end of the chapter). I decided to bite the bullet, however, and sign up.

The company gave us a list of volunteers who had signed up to go on the trip and a few of us made contact with each other before we left. I was excited about working with elephants in Thailand and had opted to work in a school in Cambodia, but about a week before I was due to leave, I was informed that schools were closed at the time of my trip and I would need to engage in another project, which would involve building a house. *Why did they only just know about this?* I asked myself. I was a bit disappointed and not sure that my skill set included building houses but was happy to give anything a go.

September 8th 2017

I fly directly to Bangkok to meet up with the rest of the group who are flying in today from all corners of the world. Two of our guide leaders meet me and four other women, two from the UK and two from the USA, at the airport and we are transported to a hotel in Bangkok. This is a city I have visited twice before, and I am eager to explore the Khao San Road again. On a previous trip to Thailand, where I had lost my baggage on the outgoing flight, I had shopped there for the infamous elephant pants and other clothes. It is hot, sticky, busy and just as I remembered, and luckily our hotel is conveniently located just around the corner from here.

For the first time, I have opted to share a room with a stranger and have some real anxieties about this with the obvious toilet issues around my Crohn's and the implications of sharing facilities. I arrive first and anxiously pace about the room. My roommate, Jackie, arrives and finds me wringing my hands. As soon as she walks into the room, I find myself telling her about my

Crohn's and say that she may wish to share with someone else. Jackie is totally understanding and, as luck would have it, tells me she is a pharmacist and understands my dilemma and is not fazed by my concerns. Jackie hails from South Africa but now lives in Vancouver. I will never forget her response today. She is more concerned about the fact that our twin beds are situated so close together than my toilet dilemma and suggests we move them a tad so we will not be breathing in each other's faces. I am relieved and we do this. One of the other volunteers texts me: *Hey… it's Darren here… just added you… am heading for some lunch in a min if you wanna join me…* We go to meet him down in the lobby and venture out for some street food and, of course, the ubiquitous foot massage… the first of many to come. Darren tells us that he is an Australian, currently living in Bahrain, and a manager of the Royal Palace. Time passes and we enjoy the buzz of the Khao San Road as the afternoon turns into evening. Jet lag is catching up with me, but it is well after midnight before we go to bed.

The next morning, we meet the rest of the party of volunteers, and I see a blonde girl with an enormous smile on her face. She introduces herself as Leesa and her two friends are Deb and Kim, all from Queensland, Australia. I learn later that they decided to embark on this adventure as they all sadly lost their husbands quite recently and are members of a widows' group back home. Our guide introduces herself again and says this is pronounced "pan" like a saucepan or a piece of bread in French. We are given a brief description about what we will be doing when we arrive at our homestay. We are told that the elephants have all been rescued from the cities where they have been used to entertain tourists and are now part of a project where families are paid a small amount to look after them and that our help will contribute to this project and the community. I am trying to envisage how such big animals can be kept in someone's back yard.

But first we have a free day and evening to visit some sights in Bangkok. First of all, we take a boat to the Taling Chan floating market, and this is where I first learn of Darren's intense love of food and photographing it! We taste all sorts of divine and extraordinary things, and this is when I have to begin to explain to my travel mates the perils of me swallowing some food which won't pass through my restricted bowel! Leaving the market behind, we visit the temples of Wat Arun and Wat Pho, which houses the enormous reclining golden Buddha. Apparently, this image represents the entry of Buddha into Nirvana and the end of all reincarnations. The figure is fifteen metres high and forty-six metres long, and it is one of the largest Buddha statues in Thailand. I've seen it twice before! This takes me back to my first visit to Bangkok with my daughter in 2003, after the Bali bombing the year before, where tourism had been affected in this part of the world. It had been very quiet at that time with a slight drizzle. This time it is hot and humid! Leesa has a "moment" and feels a bit dizzy, possibly through low blood pressure, and she needs to sit down to recover, so we think it is time to head back soon.

We take a tuk-tuk back to the hotel, where we are told we can visit a nearby hotel with a pool. I don my costume and a floaty sarong and join the others at the reception desk to walk to the hotel. Our guide tells me quite firmly that I can't walk through the streets wearing this, as it is see-through! I saw some weird sights on the Khao San Road last night, so I am unsure why she is being so prim, but I agree and find something else to wear. Our guides tell us that they are going to take us out for "one night in Bangkok", so after our swim, we get changed and off we go to the Roof Bar on the Khao San Road, where we are promised live music and Thai beer. We get to know our fellow travellers a bit better, and I even manage a dance with a young man who lets me wear his baseball cap for a while. The evening ends with a meander through the bustling Khao San Road, where Jackie and I try on skirts and elephant pants and some of the others try some delicacies, including spiders. There is no shortage of fried bugs here, but I settle for an ice cream as I am not sure how that would travel through my poor bowel.

The next day, we head north to Surin, a northern province of Thailand. One of the guides is a bit worse for wear after too many beers last night and at one point I think she is sick into her handbag. I prepare myself for a long bus journey with no toilet facilities, something which always makes me anxious. I brief our guides and explain that I may have to ask the driver to pull over at short notice. I always carry supplies of toilet paper, wet wipes and hand gel, which is doubly important in a country like this where toilet paper is not automatically supplied and the order of the day is often a squat toilet or a "squatty potty", as it is nicknamed. I often find these a bit of a challenge but over time have developed strong leg muscles for squatting and balancing. I'm not sure how people with dodgy knees manage in this situation. As it happens, this is not necessary on this occasion, and we stop several times on the way. When we are almost at our destination, our bus breaks down and we spend some time sitting on the roadside and chatting to the local police before it is fixed and we are finally on our way.

We arrive at our accommodation in the evening. I am not really sure where we are, but we seem to be in the middle of nowhere. I discover that we are in the area of Ta Thum. We are told there is a surprise for us and we clamber into a truck and head up the road to see a baby elephant. Again, we are reminded that this is a wonderful project that helps get street begging elephants out of the cities and back to a more natural setting, where they can bond as family groups and wander without chains, whilst at the same time providing a sustainable source of income for the mahouts and their families. The elephant is indeed very cute and rolls around on the floor, but we are a bit concerned that the mother elephant and her baby seem to be confined in a pen. It is explained to us that elephants can't be free to rampage around, and I suppose that is true, but I begin to wonder about their actual freedom, although I can see that for safety reasons they have to be chained up.

We go back to unpack at our accommodation, which is loosely described as an elephant village. I am sleeping in a dormitory with Jackie and two others. We have two single beds at the end of the room with covers with ducks on that look extremely grubby. We are to share a mosquito net and a fan. I can see this will be quite interesting in the middle of the night for the frequent toilet visits I have to make! I go to investigate the toilet situation and find them outside. There are no flushing toilets but there is a lot of water available for pouring into them to get rid of the contents somehow. The showers are also inside the toilet cubicles and are cold water only. I find lots of bits of old soap from previous volunteers I guess and some toothbrushes they have left behind. Darren, as the only single man, is busy acquiring some extra fans for his single room and we joke with him that there are no scatter cushions here!

We are to eat in a communal area and told that there will be a vegetarian option each night. My heart sinks a bit, and I know this is going to be a challenge for me as I often can't eat either a meat or vegetarian option due to the content. I have given a long list of foodstuffs that I will be unable to risk, especially as we appear to be far from anywhere and I haven't asked whether there is a hospital nearby. It reads like this: "Hi! Here is the list. No pork, beef or lamb. No nuts, mushrooms, dried fruit or anything with a skin. Some veg difficult if they are fibrous. No beansprouts, no coconut, no tea or coffee. Anything which is difficult to digest as I have a large part of my bowel removed. Can eat fish, chicken, prawns, rice and noodles!"

We are told that we will be making our own breakfast in the morning (cooking facilities are very limited) and that we will need to clear up, which is all good until we see the state of the kitchen, which needs a good clean. Darren gets to work! He is good at this! On the door there is a timetable of activities, and we see that there are a few sessions listed for cutting plant food for the elephants, two occasions when we will walk with the elephants and something which says "poo paper" and "building project". We are all looking forward to whatever this project brings but go to bed fairly early. Not a lot else to do really! As I expected, the trips to the loo in the night are interesting, as it is tricky to get out from under the mozzie net without tangling it up in the fan. It is a hot and sticky night. The fan moves between us, and I find myself willing it to move towards me more quickly to have a blast of air. Luckily, I don't need to cover myself up with the grubby covers.

Breakfast is disappointing the next morning, and we are given a few loaves of bread to make toast. We vow to ask for eggs the next morning. I find the guides sitting on the floor in a room outside tucking into a feast of Thai food and feel a bit miffed. How are we supposed to build up our strength for cutting down the elephant grass? We set off sometime in the middle of the day in the searing heat and are given machetes for cutting down the elephant grass. We have to slash at it and then carry large armfuls back to the truck. We need enough to feed at least twenty large elephants the next day! The work is physically exhausting and the heat and humidity very draining. It is mega-hard work, and I realise I am pretty useless at the actual cutting of the grass so opt to carry it to the truck instead. I drink lots of water but feel dehydrated after a while. This is also a common thing that happens to me because of my frequent toilet visits. I sit in the truck for a few minutes and marvel at my co-workers, who are enthusiastically hacking at the grass as if they were born to do this. One of the volunteers, Marcia, has sensibly brought with her a towel to go round her neck, which she keeps wet with cold water. Eventually, our leaders deem that we have enough food for the elephants. Really? We eat, lie in hammocks, chat and laugh for the remainder of the day.

The next day, we are to meet our elephants; the mahouts will bring them to us and we get to "choose" the elephant we will walk to the river with. I somehow end up with two, a big mummy elephant with a baby who I am told is called Rambo. We set off to walk to the river and I am holding a piece of string with Rambo on the end of it. I am also wearing flip-flops. Should Rambo decide to run off, I am not sure that string will be very effective, but the mahout seems to have everything under control. Eventually we reach the river, and this is where we all need to get in and wash the elephants. I hadn't bargained for Rambo's extreme excitement. He dashed in and started flailing and rolling around and spraying water from his little trunk. Despite the fact that he is a baby, he has large feet, and I can only guess at how much he weighs and what would happen to my foot if he stood on it. My flip-flops are sinking into the deep mud, and I am doing a lot of flailing and floundering around myself, trying to stay upright and dodge the cascade of water from Rambo's trunk. I look across at some of the others who seem to be having a calmer time of it, but I gamely try to wash my baby elephant. He is doing a pretty good job of it himself, splashing and rolling on his back. I feel I must capture this moment and try to take videos on my phone. Eventually we all start the walk home where we are to feed the elephants with the grass we gathered yesterday. The grass that had taken us hours to cut down was demolished in minutes. Logistically, I am wondering how they eat the rest of the time when we are not around, but I don't seem to come up with any answers. We are all quite muddy, so we wash ourselves off with cold water and put Darren into a barrel where we hose him down. He seems to enjoy it as much as the elephants! After this we head to the river and are instructed to collect some weed-like stuff and realise this is how we are going to learn how to make paper out of elephant poo. We join in the process and then purchase some bookmarks and books, which were made earlier by some other people, as souvenirs.

We are furnished with eggs the next morning, so Darren whips up an omelette or two. After this, we are taken kayaking. One of the kayaks sinks and once again I wonder about the health and safety aspects of this trip. Luckily, the couple in this particular kayak are experienced and manage not to drown. We set off to the fields to plant elephant grass, which involves a lot of digging dry earth. Without being too cynical, I am wondering if anything will really get planted here. We ponder on why we were kayaking early and cutting grass afterwards and I sense a mutiny. We ask if we could please do the more exhausting work earlier in the morning when it is not so darned hot! It crosses my mind that we are all of a certain age and I wonder whether these young leaders are trained in first aid or CPR. One of us could have a heart attack and this is not beyond the realms of possibility. We do our best with the grass and in the evening we go to a local market where we buy some local foodstuffs to help eke out our rather meagre and repetitive diet.

Thursday dawns and it seems that we have to cut more elephant food for their last visit tomorrow but also engage in a building project. We drive to a field and are told that we are going to start to make a pig pen. I haven't seen any pigs anywhere. I kind of feel that this is just to keep us busy and struggle with digging holes into the dry earth. I find myself standing with my arms folded surveying the scene and frowning. One or two people are putting all of their energy into digging these holes. I really just can't see the point and think there is no pig pen and that they will just fill in the holes when we have left. Call me cynical… hmmmm.

The next day is our last day with the elephants, and we are now old hands and know what to expect. I put on some better footwear for a start. I put on the wet shoes my daughter lent me, and I fear that once they have been in the stinking mud they won't be leaving the elephant village in my bag. We walk to the river and I try to avoid being squashed by Rambo. He is very cute though. I now find myself dwelling on this project and whether these elephants are indeed happy or not. Are we being conned here? Am I contributing to the use of elephants for tourism in the guise of volunteering? I have seen them rocking from side to side on their chains and it takes me back to a time when I was in Sri Lanka at the Kandy Perahera, which is a pageant involving elephants. I recall feeling extremely uncomfortable watching the elephants moving through the streets and rocking from side to side. How could they be coping with the thunderous noise of the crowds, the burning torches and the flashing lights, not to mention the fact that I had seen them tethered in the city during the day. I feel discombobulated and sad remembering that evening and thinking of these elephants here.

Our experience in Surin is over and the next day we clean the area and prepare to leave to cross the border into Cambodia for the next part of the volunteer experience. After another long bus journey, I am quite desperate for the toilet, but my fellow travellers are getting used to me disappearing with very little notice. We cross at the O Smach/Chong Chom border, which is relatively easy, and head towards Siem Reap which is 150km away. Our guide warned us several times that we will find this country very dirty and full of rubbish on the streets. We can see already that she is right.

Our bus pulls into the drive of our hotel, which is called Le Watwam Hotel, and we feel very excited as we spy a swimming pool and a massive amount of food spread out to greet us on our arrival. *This is more like it*, I am ashamed to think. Jackie and I have a room overlooking the pool with twin beds and our own bathroom and a flushing toilet. Luxury!

That night, we get into a tuk-tuk and head into town. Siem Reap is busy and we go to the infamous Pub Street, which is full of lively bars and restaurants. What I really want is a foot massage and there are countless places offering this service. We don't loiter too late, as we are going to get up very early so that we can make our way to Angkor Wat to see the sun rise. It is rumoured that the sun comes up behind the largest spire and is a sight not to be missed.

It is dark when we get up and we collect a packed lunch and climb into tuk-tuks. It is raining very hard, although it is hot. Somehow it all goes wrong and there is some misunderstanding about the collection of our tickets. By the time we arrive, we have missed the sunrise and the rain is heavy. A guide has been organised to tell us about the history of Angkor Wat, but we are not very good students and several of us wander off to look at and photograph the temple. We are making a day of it and visit Bayon, Angkor Thom and Ta Prohm where *Tomb Raider* was filmed. I think this is my favourite, with its crumbling towers, doorways and the weirdest trees and roots I have ever seen. We have our photo taken by the "*Tomb Raider* tree". It is a great day and eventually the rain eases off and we head back to our hotel for a dip in the pool.

The next day we are to start our next volunteer project. As a few of us had expressed disappointment about not going to visit a school, a visit has been arranged for the morning. We set off in tuk-tuks to Slarkram English School, where we are given information about the school, which provides free English classes to the rural children from the village nearby. These children would otherwise barely learn any English or even receive any education at all. We are shown donations of clothes and big bags of rice and then we get dispatched to a classroom. Jackie and I go as a pair, and we have a lot of fun working with the children, who are delightful and so well behaved. They find us funny and there is a lot of laughter. It makes me smile to see the classroom rules displayed on the wall in English. Number ten is "have fun and be safe".

We learn that the school is part of a project called New Hope, which provides free education, free healthcare, and crisis and community support for children and young people who come from the nearby village of Mondul Bei. There is also a training restaurant as part of this, which aims to teach unemployed and uneducated young people cooking and hospitality skills and develop their confidence and employment opportunities. We eat our lunch here before heading into the village of Mondul 3.

The next hour of so becomes pretty surreal. We are given black plastic bags and tasked with the job of cleaning up rubbish in the village. There is so much rubbish it is unbelievable. We are not given any plastic gloves. A lot of villagers and small children and skinny cats sit around in the sun watching us. There are some small shops selling, it seems, mainly nappies and sweets. This feels like another particularly strange use of our time. How is this going to help the villagers long-term, watching a group of strangely clad Westerners cleaning up their rubbish? Again, it feels as if they are just filling our time with useless activities on this project.

After a short time, we leave the village and get into our minibus to head for the destination where we are about to embark on our major project, which involves tearing down a house and building a more substantial one for a family. Our first job is to completely dismantle the existing dwelling. We have no gloves and no goggles to protect our hands and eyes. We try our hardest but ask if we can at least be provided with some form of protection, so one of the staff sets off on a bike and returns with some plastic gloves. After a couple of hours, the bamboo hut which has housed this family is in bits on the floor. End of day one! I wonder where they will sleep tonight? We can't wait to get back to the hotel, shower thoroughly and get into the pool, which makes me reflect on how fortunate we are, and I feel a little guilty.

The next day, after breakfast, we leave early and start the task of building the new house for the family. Some locals and a contractor have been brought in to help with laying the foundations and some brick work. We are shown how to whittle down bamboo sticks and make a frame by nailing wood together. Banana leaves then have to be painstakingly stuck together with wire to make the sides of the house and the roof. It's hard work in the heat and we work diligently until lunchtime when we are taken off to the Fat Panda Café for lunch and, in the afternoon, back to the same tasks. Some of us are better at it than others. I am impressed by Leesa and Jackie's ability to nail things together. I find myself with several others tying the bamboo leaves onto what will be the sides of the house. At one point, I lie on the floor to get a better grip and realise that I have put my head in some dog poo. I go to the squat toilet in an empty building next to where we are working and try to wash it off. I stink! This is the toilet I have to use if I need to during the day. Cambodians with little money do not use toilet paper, so lots of cold water has to suffice. Luckily, in this heat you dry off quickly!

Over the next couple of days, things begin to take shape, and it is an exciting moment when the roof gets put on to the walls and it actually looks like a house, a much more substantial one than the one the family had lived in before. The floor is yet to be completed and will be put in later… hopefully! We club together to equip the house with some basics and Darren goes off in a tuk-tuk and returns laden with pots, pans, bed coverings, mattresses and all sorts of things. The family are thrilled, and we all pose for a photo in front of the house. Their faces and their gratitude make all of the hard work worthwhile and put into perspective my worries about going to the toilet. Our project is finished!

We celebrate that night by going to the Red Piano in Pub Street, which is where Angelina Jolie allegedly hung out when she was filming *Tomb Raider*. There is even a *Tomb Raider* cocktail, which is made of lime juice, Cointreau and tonic! It's a fun place and we are in high spirits. This is our last night together as a group, as tomorrow we will all be heading in different directions. We are elated but sad that the experience is over. We have had such fun, laughing every day, and I know that I will most definitely be seeing the Aussie trio (Leesa, Deb and Kim) and Darren and Jackie again!

The next morning, we say our goodbyes and I head off on a bus to Phnom Penh, as I am extending my tour and spending another week in Cambodia. Ravy is with me as my guide, and we board a bus and prepare for a long journey south. I read my guidebook and learn a bit more about Cambodia's troubled history. I cannot do it justice here, but I can't write this chapter without making some reference to it.

In brief, the Khmer Rouge was a brutal regime that ruled Cambodia under the leadership of Marxist dictator Pol Pot from 1975 to 1979. He gained power and instituted a radical reorganisation of Cambodian society, attempting to create a Cambodian "master race" through social engineering. This meant the forced removal of city dwellers into the countryside, where they would be compelled to work as farmers, digging canals and tending to crops. Gross mismanagement of the country's economy led to shortages of food and medicine, and untold numbers of people succumbed to disease and starvation. Families were also split up. The Khmer Rouge created labour brigades, assigning groups depending on age and gender. This policy resulted in hundreds of thousands of Cambodians starving to death.

Religious and ethnic minorities faced particular persecution. Christian and Buddhist groups were targeted for repression, but it was the Cham Muslim group that was most affected by the genocide. As many as 500,000 people, or seventy per cent of the total Cham population, were exterminated. Because the Khmer Rouge placed a heavy emphasis on the rural peasant population, anyone considered an intellectual was targeted for special treatment. This meant teachers, lawyers, doctors, and clergy were the targets of the regime. Even people wearing glasses were the target of Pol Pot's reign of terror.

There is difficulty establishing a definitive number of victims of the Cambodian Genocide. The Cambodians kept methodical records of prisoners and executions. However, because Cambodia's enemy, Vietnam, invaded and released the records, there is speculation they could have been exaggerated. In addition, estimating the total number of people who starved is difficult. Estimates range from 1.5 to three million people having died at the hands of the Khmer Rouge, with the consensus being approximately two million.

So, here I am on a bus heading towards Phnom Penh, where I am booked in for a couple of nights at the Paragon Hotel. I check in and Ravy shows me around parts of the city. I get the feeling that he is not too familiar with it. I don't think he has been given much of a budget to feed himself by the company either. We head towards the Royal Palace and then walk about the city. It feels very different from Siem Reap and, indeed, it is much bigger. The streets are filled with rubbish and there is a lot of traffic with many tuk-tuks, cars and motorcycles.

The next day, we go by tuk-tuk to the Tuol Sleng Genocide Museum, also known as S-21. It was originally a secondary school but between the years of 1975–1979 it served as a secret facility for the detention, interrogation, torture and extermination of those deemed "political enemies" of the regime. An estimated twenty thousand people were imprisoned here. Due to a policy of guilt-by-association, at times whole families were detained at the centre. There are four blocks, with cells containing iron bedsteads, shackles, instruments of torture and hundreds of photographs of the victims. It is a harrowing place to visit and eerily silent. I walk round alone and reflect on what I had been doing in the UK during these years. This was at the height of the punk era, where people were free to express themselves in whatever manner they chose. The contrast is stark. I come outside into the sunshine where I meet Chum Mey, one of only seven adult survivors from this dark place. He is selling copies of his book. *Survivor: The Triumph of an Ordinary Man in The Khmer Rouge Genocide*. I sit next to him and try to speak but my eyes are filled with tears. He doesn't speak much English but there is someone nearby who translates. How did he survive? He was a mechanic who could mend sewing machines so somehow he was spared. We hug each other and I think to myself he has such a kind face. For once in my life, I have no words. I can barely speak to Ravy when we leave and wonder how he must be feeling and how many in his own family have suffered.

We move on to the next destination, which is equally as harrowing, if not more, somehow. This is Choeung Ek Killing Fields. Apart from when I visited Dachau in Germany and Auschwitz in Poland, I have never had such an unpleasant feeling flood my whole being. The atmosphere is suffocating. I find it hard to read the details of what happened here, and I can't write about it and do it justice. I am told that the Cambodians are transparent; they provide a non-sanitised account of their recent history and are active even in broadcasting all that happened in the hope that it will never happen again anywhere in the world. If you haven't been and want to know about it, then I will leave you to do your own research.

The next day, Ravy and I catch another bus and head further south to Sihanoukville on the coast, where we arrive in the rain in the darkness. I meet up with Marina, who has also made her way here from the project, and she is pleased to see a familiar face. She is staying in Serendipity Beach, so I plan to go there in the morning to explore the area.

In the morning, Ravy and I hire a motorbike and go to meet up with Marina. We ride along the coastline to Otres Beach and Independence Beach. All I can say is that it doesn't look good. This place used to be popular with backpackers as a boho hippie hangout but is now being taken over by Chinese companies constructing massive hotels. There are half-built hotels everywhere and the noise of construction fills your ears. I am trying to imagine what this place will look like in a couple of years, and it is not a nice image. It is also extremely dirty, and we don't fancy our chances in the sea, which is full of rubbish and plastic bags. It's a fun outing though and the next day we plan to get a boat over to the island of Koh Rong Sanloem. In a travel guide, this island is described as "a peaceful relaxing destination with breath-taking scenery – pristine white beaches, clear turquoise ocean waters, and a tropical jungle wilderness. A real 'island paradise'." I look forward to this!

I wake up to the kind of rain that you only see in other countries, or sometimes in Wales. Not to be deterred, we don some waterproofs and swimming gear and head to the boat. When we arrive at the island, the sun comes out and it is a lovely day and a fine end to my trip. I lie on the sand and reflect on my experiences in these countries. Tomorrow, I will take the bus back to Phnom Penh, where I will stay for just one more night and then fly home to the UK with my head full of the experiences I have had over the last few weeks and some amazing brand-new friends scattered across the globe. I can't wait to catch up with them to see what adventures they have had since leaving the project. Last but not least, I survived the adventure despite my Crohn's disease!

There is just one more hurdle to overcome. I return by bus to Phnom Penh and the Paragon Hotel, where I am greeted like an old friend. Ravy waves goodbye as he is heading back to Siem Reap. In the morning, I wake up and pack my bags for the last time on this trip. I go into the hotel lobby to wait for the tuk-tuk driver, who brought us here a week or so ago and had arranged to pick me up to take me to the airport. The driver arrives and announces that he is the brother of my arranged driver and that he is replacing him. He appears to be completely drunk. He grabs my bags and heads out of the hotel to put them into the tuk-tuk. The person on the reception desk is looking worried and has summoned the manager. They tell me that it is not wise to go with this man in his tuk-tuk. I agree but am not sure what I will do as I need to get to the airport.

"I will take you!" announces the manager.

Firstly, we have to retrieve my bags. The tuk-tuk driver is not pleased. There is a lot of shouting! I stand

and watch the hotel staff grappling with the driver and wrenching my bags from the back of the tuk-tuk. He gives in and leaves yelling and swearing. An air-conditioned car miraculously arrives, and I am ushered inside. Another disaster averted. I lean back and look around me as we head towards the airport, and I have to say that I am glad I am not in that tuk-tuk. Goodbye, Cambodia!

After returning home, some of the group who had participated in the volunteer project decided to contact the sales and customer operations director of the company. Three of the group sent long emails, outlining concerns and giving them some feedback on our experiences. Darren also offered a financial donation to help with the elephant project and the school fees for the child of the family for whom we built the house. This offer was not followed up by the company. We received a response to our emails, however, and we were promised that the areas we had highlighted would be addressed and changes implemented. That is all we could have hoped for, I suppose.

Footnote: What Happened to the Company?

The company folded in 2022 and newspaper articles available on the internet give the reasons why. Would-be tourists who lost thousands say the director and co-founder "have been living lavishly with 'extravagant' weddings, overseas holidays and a plan to build a boat and sail the world". A liquidation report revealed that one of the directors put more than US$2 million of customer funds into multiple cryptocurrency platforms from October 2020 until mid 2022 and lost all of the money. Hundreds of customers who had already paid for their holidays would not be receiving refunds under the "force majeure" section of the terms and conditions. In a statement at the time of the closure, the company blamed Covid and a small group of customers who weren't prepared to wait for refunds. Many customers were also caught out after buying a Chubb travel insurance package through the company's website, only to be told by Chubb their insurance was not valid.

This boat-building project is documented on the director's Facebook page, along with posts about international holidays, including a trip to Thailand in mid 2022, just months before the company announced its closure. The page still exists but the last post on his page is from June 2022.

This was the statement issued by the company online:

"This is a tough one. The beautiful dream can no longer continue. Through the challenges of COVID and a looming recession, we thought we had found a way to keep the journey going. For 10+ years, we have strived to share our love of travel and how it can be a force of positivity in the world. With deep regret and due to reasons beyond our ability to control, we advise that '*the company*' has reluctantly ceased to operate. If you are a customer of '*the company*' please get in touch with us with the email address provided at booking. If you have ever experienced a tour and wish to post your best memories with us as a review, it would be greatly received. Although we no longer operate, and this site no longer serves as a marketing tool, we still recognize the many thousands who have possibly changed their lives and the lives of others through our give-back adventures."

You can draw your own conclusions. I feel very sorry for all of the people who put their trust in these people and lost their money. I also feel a bit foolish that I was taken in by their false promises about the worthiness of their projects. I wonder what has happened to the people who worked for them, the local people we met and, of course, the elephants. I am still occasionally in touch with Ravy, who worked for them and accompanied me to the south of the country as a guide. I sent some money over to him for his family during Covid, as I was aware that he had lost his job with the company.

At the end of the day, however, I had the pleasure of travelling in these countries and meeting the most amazing group of people who shared this journey with me and who I know will be friends for life. In addition, my guide Ravy and I are still in touch and I recently set up a GoFundMe page to help him to further his career in teaching and attend and speak at a recent teacher development conference in Vietnam.

Twelve

Trekking in the Mountains of Albania and Transylvania to Raise Money for Crohn's

2018

Apart from volunteering last September in Thailand and Cambodia, my last challenge was the big one last year trekking in Peru to raise money for forCrohn's. In July, I will be taking on another challenge raising money for the charity, climbing three peaks in Transylvania in three days. As I need to be as fit as possible for this, I decide to take a holiday in Albania walking in the mountains in the north of the country. This is also part of my "mission" to travel to more places off the beaten track to see how easy (or difficult) it is to travel with Crohn's disease.

Albania has only really opened up to tourism in the last five years. I imagine that the south and the beach areas are more geared up for tourists than the area I was visiting in the north.

I leave to fly via Vienna. Of course, aeroplanes are a particular challenge with limited toilet facilities which often have queues. I always ask for an aisle seat but when the hostesses bring the refreshments tray down the aisle, it is difficult to access them without climbing over the trolley, which isn't popular! Short flights aren't so bad but of course Crohn's is never predictable, and you can't plan your toilet visits.

Arriving at the airport near Tirana, I am picked up and join a group of fifteen people I have never met before for a two-hour drive in a minibus to the town of Shkodra, known as the capital of northern Albania. Straight away, I explain to the guide that I may ask to stop on the way and, of course, he has never heard of Crohn's disease and looks blank. I sit up at the front with him and take the opportunity to tell him what I can and can't eat and what may happen if I eat something I shouldn't. He looks a bit nonplussed.

We look around Rozafa Castle and I get to know my fellow walkers a bit better at dinner. The next morning, we drive through stunning mountain scenery to the docks at Lake Koman, where we take a ferry ride for two hours. This is described in the *Bradt* guide as "one of the world's classic boat trips" and it does not disappoint. The boat glides through glassy emerald-green waters and the twists and turns of narrow waterways beneath stunning mountain peaks. There is a toilet on the ferry, which is a relief, and although not the best, it is better than some that I have encountered around the world.

This has been the easy bit. Now we are to drive a bit further and, after lunch, begin our first walk to break us in gently. We follow the path of the river, occasionally ascending and descending. Due to the excessive rain of the winter, the river is full. Suddenly, we come to what was once a bridge across the river but unfortunately it has collapsed into the water and is impassable. Our guide tells us that there is no choice. We have to get across the river somehow as all of our luggage is heading to the next place where we are to stay the night and we can't go back, we must go forward. Our intrepid guides find a tree trunk which has fallen partly across the river and suggest that we walk across in single file. This looks a bit risky, but it seems we have no choice. There is a fast-flowing torrent beneath us. A makeshift branch "handrail" is found, and the two guides hold each end and encourage us to cross. I know my balance isn't great so we ask if we can throw our rucksacks across. They agree and we totter across and all make it safely to the other side. No risk assessments in Albania!

I have been feeling quite well recently but my three-monthly B12 could not be squeezed in before this trip, so my energy levels are low. I am not sure yet how physically tough this is going to be, but I have some worries about my ability to do it. I also realise as we move further northwards that we have left any chance of a hospital far behind us and the infrastructure suggests that it would not be easy to access one if needed. It makes me remember my trip in Madagascar when I became ill, and I am glad that I have some medicines with me in case of emergency.

Over the next few days, we trek in the Valbona National Park in the north of the country. Valbona is based in the Tropojë District of northern Albania which, along with two adjoining districts, encompasses a region called the Malësi. Roughly translated, this means "the Highlands". This is a wild and high mountainous region, inhabited by fiercely independent and strong people who have never really been conquered or subdued by the various invasions in the last two thousand years! The full name of the mountains around Valbona are the Malësia e Gjakovës and this name is most often translated in English as "the Accursed Mountains". The temperature is slightly cooler in the mountains but still hot for walking and climbing. The scenery is spectacular and there is still a lot of snow on the peaks.

Day three arrives and we learn that we are to undertake our longest climb and need horses and mules to carry our luggage, as we will be staying over the other side of the pass. A few of us ask if we can ride over the Valbona Pass and it is agreed that we can hire some extra mules. This will give me an opportunity to enjoy the scenery without constantly looking down at my feet. We drive to the top of the valley in Rrogam, where the road ends. Here, our luggage is loaded onto horses. We mount up and set off walking uphill to reach the Valbona Springs via a steep and winding forest trail. The mule is sure-footed but as we get higher and reach the snow, it seems like a good idea to dismount. The trail has narrowed, and I am riding right near the edge. Sure-footed or not, if we are to tumble, the outcome will not be good. It is really too steep to continue on horseback and these edges are frankly terrifying.

We reach a stretch of snow which looks as if it has fallen from above, but we apparently need to cross this.

The horsemen go ahead with spades to clear a path, and the mules are to go first to flatten the path a bit more, I assume. The path is six inches wide and beneath is a sheer drop down the mountainside. My heart is in my mouth as I go across, as the thought of any of us slipping down the mountain is not one to contemplate. How would we be rescued? No mountain rescue here! We all make it safely across and continue our climb upwards. The view is breathtaking, though, when we finally reach the top.

We arrive at our destination in Theth after getting soaked by a downpour of rain, which always seems to happen at the same time in the afternoon. We are to stay in a guesthouse run by a local family who are very welcoming. The accommodation is fairly basic, and I am to share a room with three others. Twelve of us are sharing two toilets with showers so I feel a little anxious about this but ask the family who own the accommodation if there is another toilet I can use in an emergency. They may have thought this request a bit odd, but it is too difficult to explain, as my Albanian is limited to saying "thank you". It is comfortable and I sleep well but in the morning one of the others in the room complains that I have been snoring. The joys of sharing a room with strangers. I apologise but she is disgruntled and asks if she can have a different room. The answer is clear. She can't!

The last day's half-day trek proves to be the hardest for me. We are to make an ascent in the direction of the Thore Pass and it is estimated that this should take us three hours. Three of the group opt to travel in the bus with the luggage and I have to admit to being tempted but I don't succumb! It is so hard, and I find myself slipping to the back of the group, as I am so slow. At one point, I lose the rest of the party as I am somewhere in the middle and the people ahead of me have gone so far ahead that I can't see them through the forest. I use my whistle on the rucksack and the guide comes running through the trees. He is a bit cross and tells me that my whistle should only be used in an emergency. It felt like one to me, alone in the woods! As we climb on, I really feel like giving up and have these gripping pains in my stomach, meaning that I have to drop behind the group to use the "outdoor toilet". One of the members of the group holds my poles and waits for me, for which I am grateful. The fastest in the group does it in three hours and the remaining six of us manage it in three hours and fifteen minutes. The view, at the memorial of Edith Durham (known as "the Queen of the Highlands" in respect of her support of the Albanian cause after World War One), is worth it, as is the feeling of accomplishment. I feel on top of the world, literally and metaphorically.

We are then transported by minibus back to the city of Tirana where we are to end our journey with a walking tour of the city and a final meal together. This involves a four-hour minibus drive so we can rest and snooze on the way. The city of Tirana is the cultural, entertainment and political centre of Albania and home to a rapidly growing population of one million (the total population of Albania stands at around just three million). There is a strange mixture of buildings: brightly painted apartment blocks, some remaining communist buildings, a bunker, theatres, restaurants and lots of bars. As a tourist, it feels very safe and there is no hassle from anyone trying to sell you anything. In fact, I don't think we have encountered any other English people during the week.

What will stick in my mind about this trip is the hospitality and generosity of the Albanian people, the absolutely stunning scenery, and the help and support from some members of the group who were all complete strangers at the beginning of the trip. There are now fifteen more people and two explore guides who perhaps know more about Crohn's disease than they did a week ago (apart from the doctor who was a member of the group and on holiday). There were other people in the group dealing with their own physical and emotional challenges who did not manage to complete all of the climbs for one reason or another. Most of the group were supportive of each other and understanding of individual circumstances and I have found this to be the case when I travel, which gives me the confidence to do this. As always, I thank my lucky stars that I didn't need hospital treatment, and my emergency medical kit has returned with me intact this time! Fingers crossed for Transylvania.

I now have six weeks to increase my level of fitness before tackling the three peaks in Transylvania. I have so far raised almost £2000 and hope to exceed this amount before I go.

Three Peaks Challenge in Transylvania

Transylvania is probably best known for Dracula's Castle and vampires, so a lot of jokes about eating garlic were made before I set off. Oh, and of course the movie *Hotel Transylvania*, but yes, it is a real place and very beautiful it is too. It is described as a "hidden gem", and I believe that King Charles also has a soft spot for the country and has been involved in conservation projects in some of the rural villages. After the end of World War One, Transylvania was united with Romania. It is located in Central Romania about a three-and-a-half-hour drive from the city of Bucharest. Transylvania literally means "land beyond the forest" so, as expected, there are lots of trees! It is also renowned for bears but sadly, or luckily, we did not come across any in the mountains.

Following my challenging trek last April in Peru, I wanted to set myself another challenge for fundraising without the punishing addition of the altitude. One of the group who trekked in Peru was organising a Three Peaks Challenge in Transylvania, so I asked her if I could join the group. Last year, I managed to get a lot more sponsorship and arranged more fundraising events, but it is always harder the second time around.

The group comprises eight people and most of the others know each other from past experiences of walking and climbing. We meet at the airport and are transported to our accommodation, which is very different from the "wild camping" in Peru and very comfortable. I have my own room. We are located near to "Dracula's Castle" in Bran near to the Carpathian Mountains, which is the second largest mountain range in Europe.

The first day, our first ascent is to take six hours up the sacred Bucegi Mountains, the highest point of which is 2,505 metres and is believed to be the home of the divine being Zamolxis (or Zeus for local ancestors). We set off early, which is always difficult for me, as dealing with my Crohn's in the morning is usually the worst time. As we set out to climb upwards, I fall towards the back immediately and feel vaguely nauseous. Most of the group are significantly younger than me and there is thirty-six years' difference between me and the youngest member of the group. The organisers of the trip, Delia and Danny, and their friend, Cristi, who accompany us, could not be more helpful and encouraging, but I am finding it tough going and I am very slow. The weather is not especially kind, and it is raining a fair amount and is also very cold for June. At the peak it is misty, and I am glad that I have brought an extra coat but wish that I had brought gloves with me. It is hard not to think about England basking in a heatwave. We don't stay long at the top and our descent is much faster, although hard on the knees. It has been a long day but back at the chalet we are given a fantastic three-course meal of traditional Transylvanian food to build up our strength for the next day's peak.

The next day, our second peak is called the Prince's Stone Mountain, the highest point being 2,237 metres. This is the west frontier of Dracula's Valley and considered to be the most spectacular in the country. It is a natural protected park, home to the famous Carpathian black goat and the only place where you can find Prince's Gillyflower. We are told that it is a shorter climb but steeper and that it should take four hours to reach the peak. Today, I do not feel so good and have to take a lot of toilet stops, which slows me up and leaves me way behind the others. The climb is steep, and it rains on and off. Cristi is amazing and very kind and encouraging, keeping me going when I feel like giving up. When I reach the point where we have planned to stop, I am way behind the others. Two of the group are eating their lunch there but the others have opted to climb further up onto the ridge to get a better view. It is too late for us to follow them as the weather is deteriorating. I must admit that I am relieved and also aware that a lot of energy is going to be required for the descent, but at least I have reached the top. The others join us at the bottom and report that they couldn't see much from the ridge and had fallen over several times due to the rocky terrain. We are all pretty exhausted and almost everyone falls asleep on the drive back.

The next day, the third peak is not quite what I have envisaged and is a short "hike" up to Poiana Braşov up in the mountains and is a popular ski resort in the area. This feels very easy after the previous two days of hard climbing. At the "top", we are treated to a fantastic traditional Transylvanian lunch. Delia and Danny want to share more of their country with us and take us to visit "Dracula's Castle" and to the medieval town of Braşov. We learn about the story of Vlad the Impaler – the Wallachian knight depicted by Bram Stoker in his novel. In the evening, we have our last meal with some traditional dancing with local children and then we party until the early hours. We will all be leaving tomorrow but I will stay on for a couple of days in Bucharest.

This has not been quite as difficult as my experience in Peru but for me it has still been a challenge! I'm wondering whether I am more suited to walking on flat ground, perhaps in the desert? Or Norfolk. It has been a great experience with a fantastic, supportive group of people who are so much fun. No tears this time!

On another note, I have been prescribed with some new medication because it seems that I am only absorbing one per cent of bile due to the resection of the particular part of my bowel and this is contributing to the chronic diarrhoea. It seems strange that it has taken them so many years to figure this out. Who knows, maybe next year I won't be trailing along at the back, as I won't have to keep stopping and won't feel so fatigued. Fingers crossed and watch this space! What will the next challenge be?

"We did it forCrohn's" hallenge ends in Machu Picchu

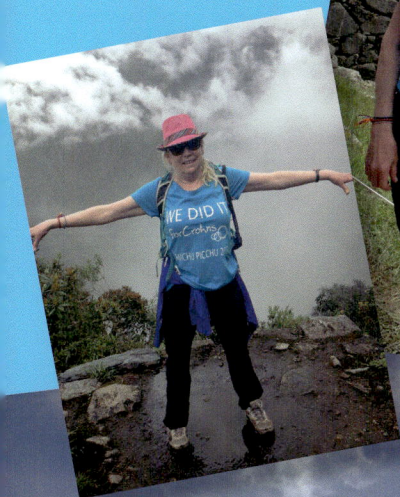

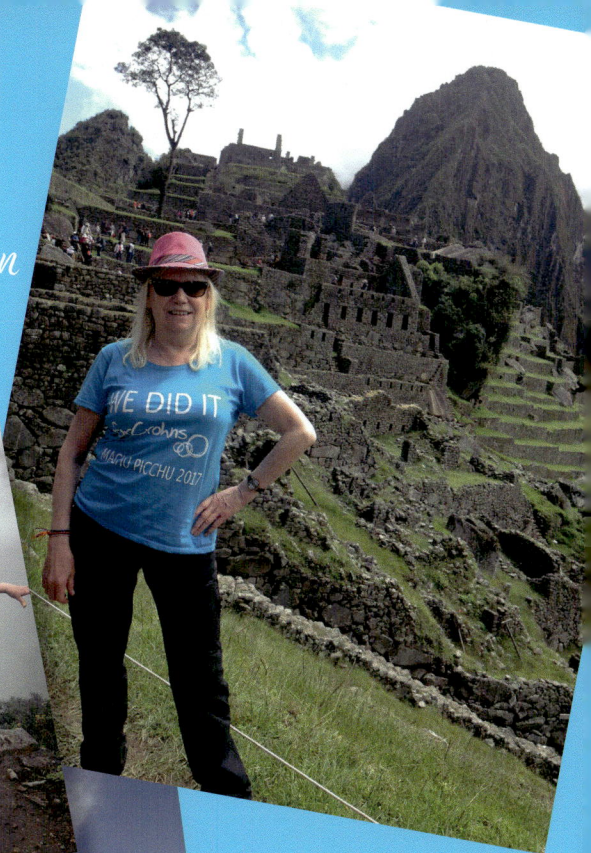

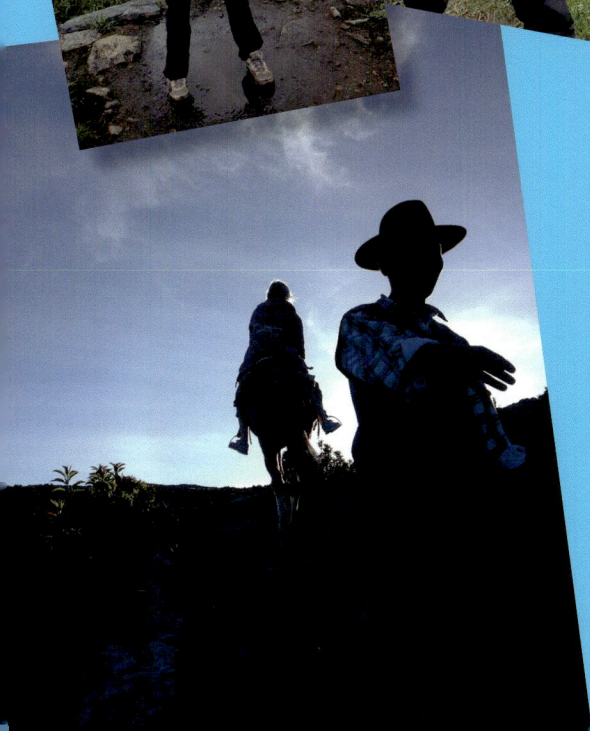

Catching the sunset on Lake Titicaca

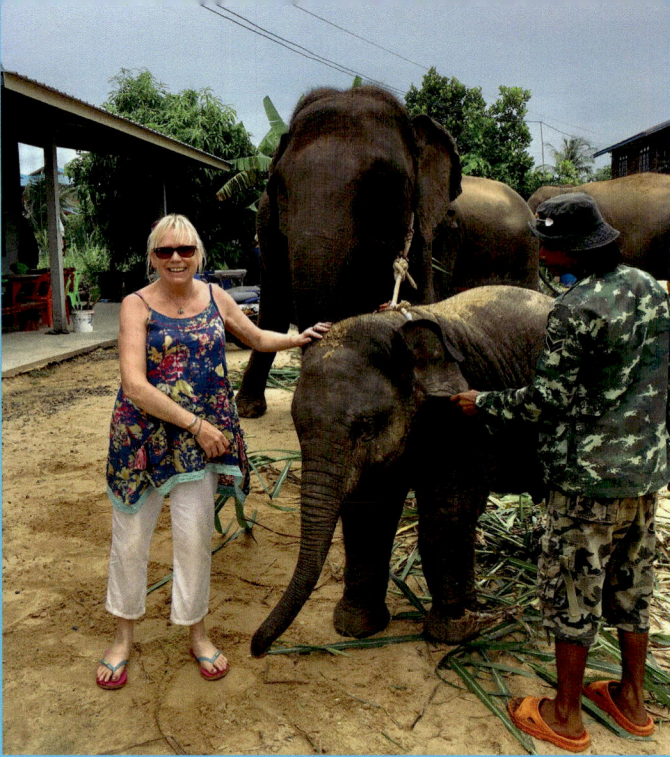

Volunteering with elephants in Thailand

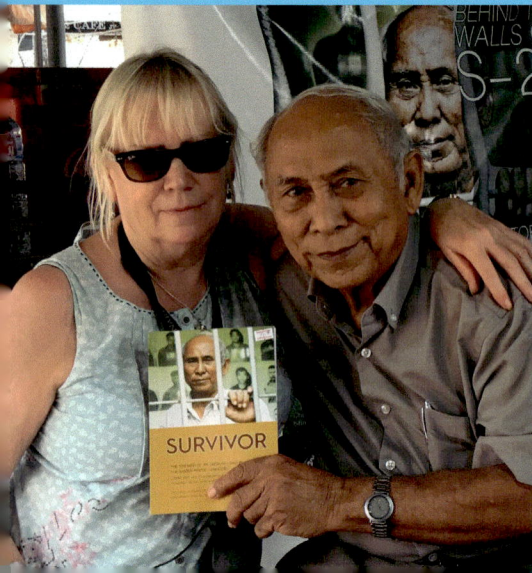

Cambodian genocide survivor from Tuol Sleng

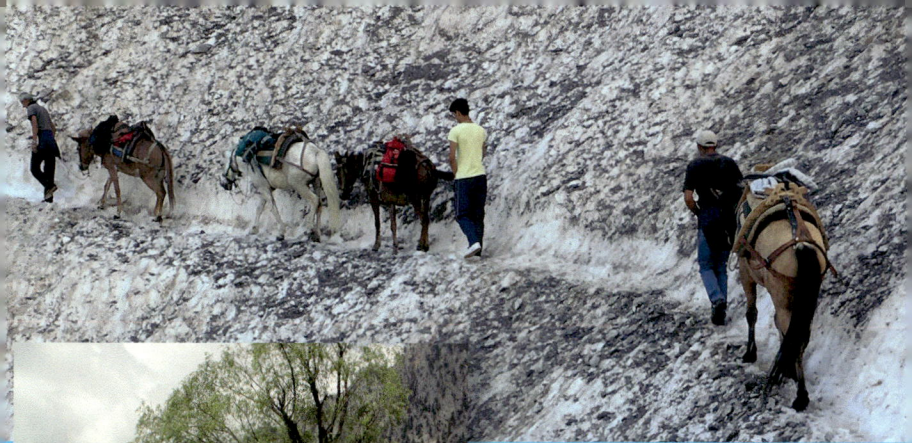

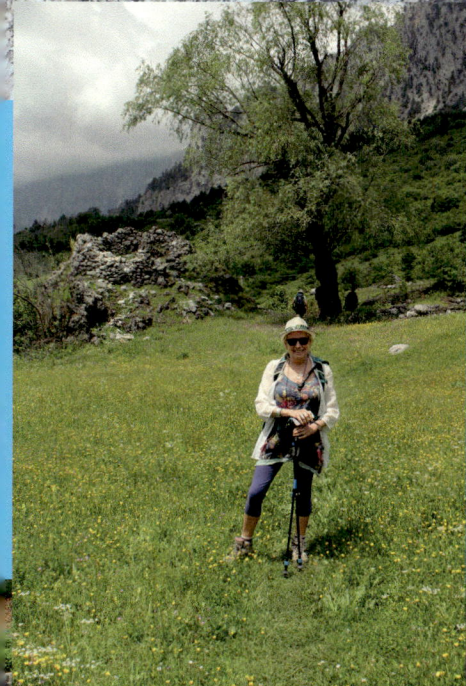

Broken bridge – some unexpected challenges in Albania

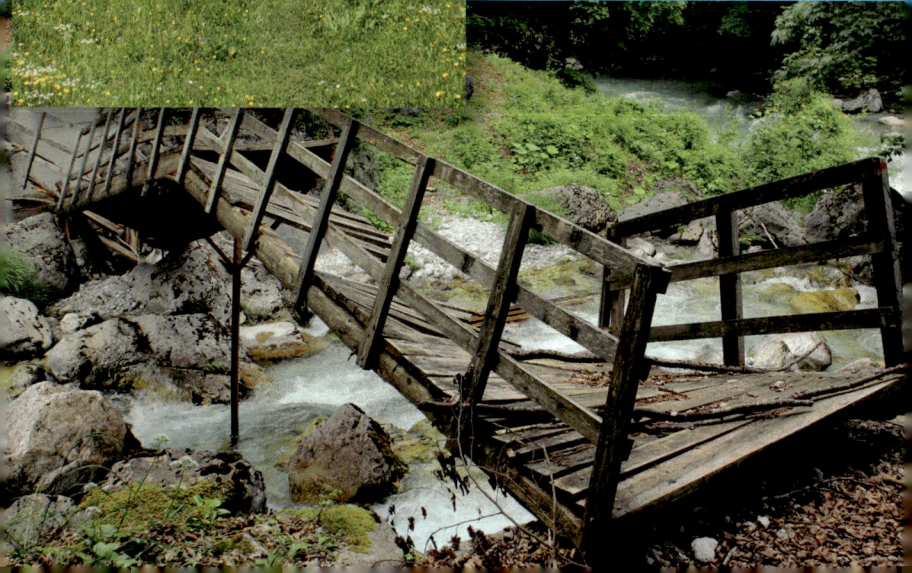

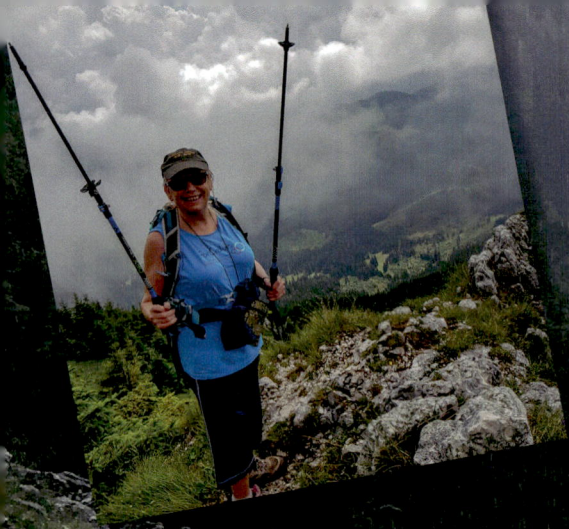

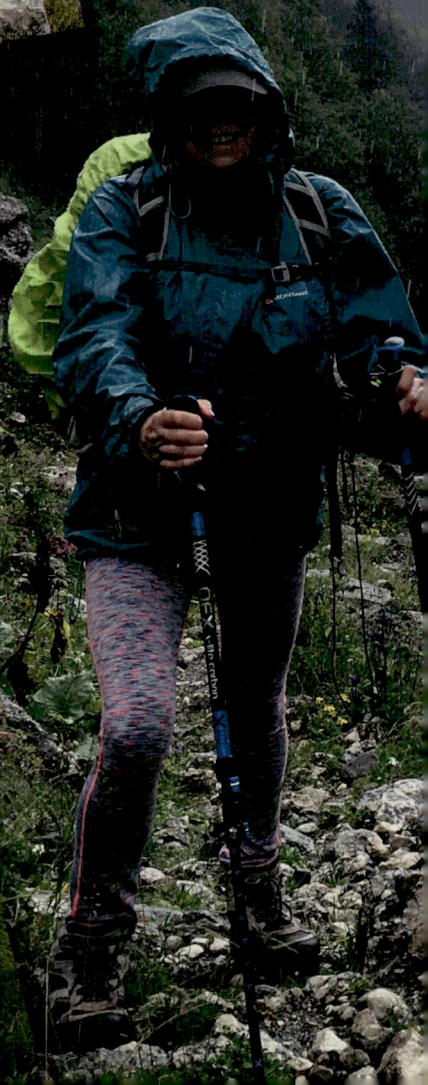

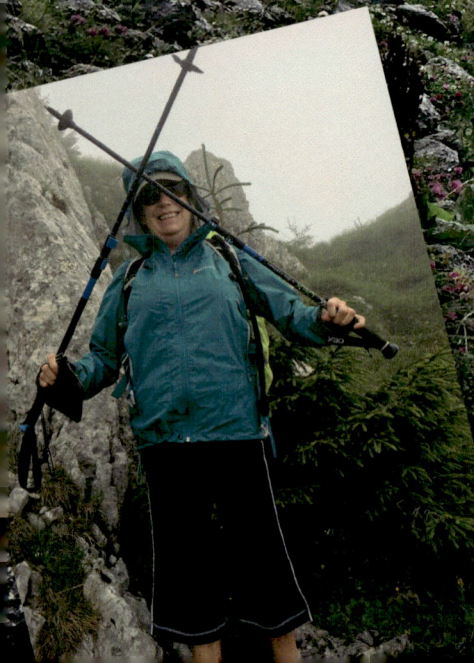

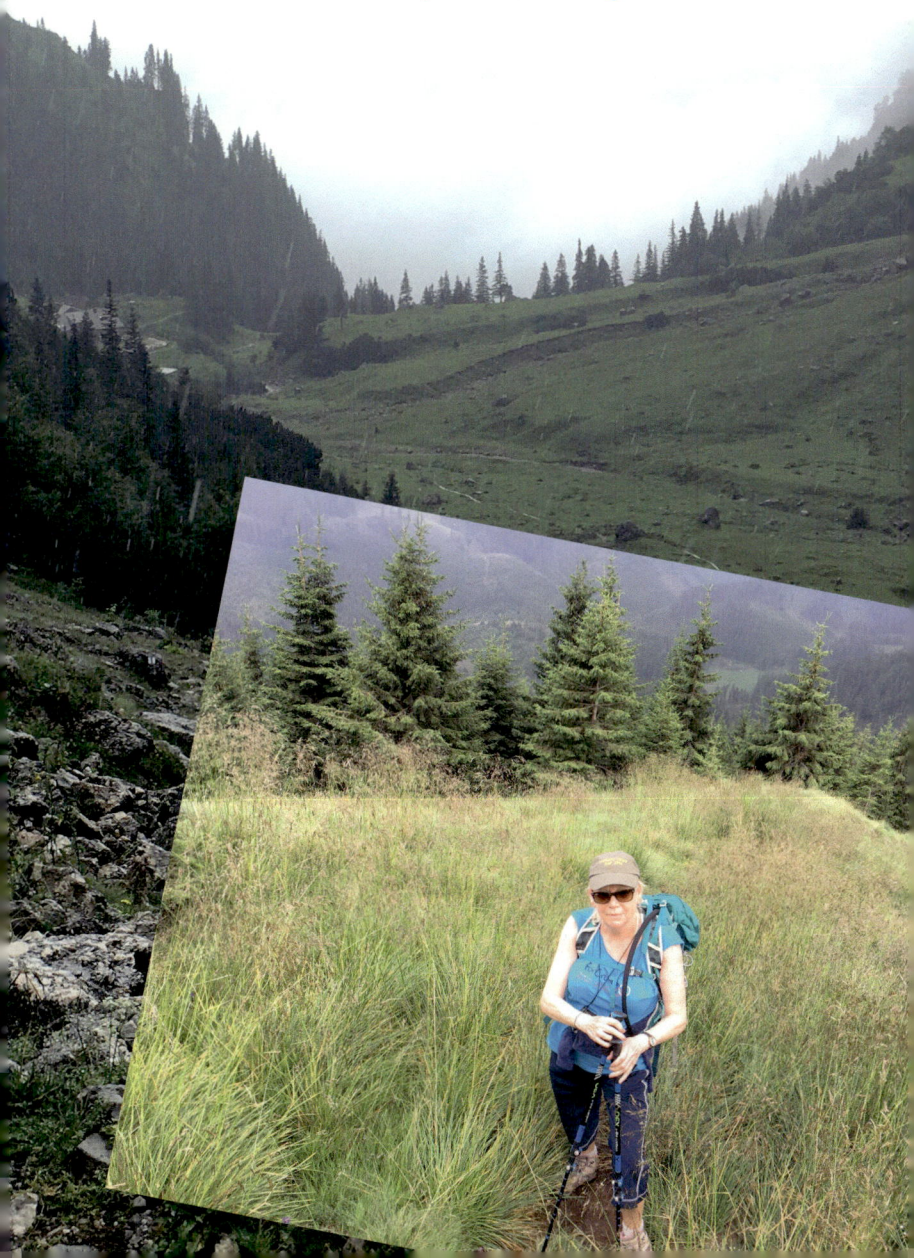

Conquering three peaks for Crohn's – fundraising in Transylvania

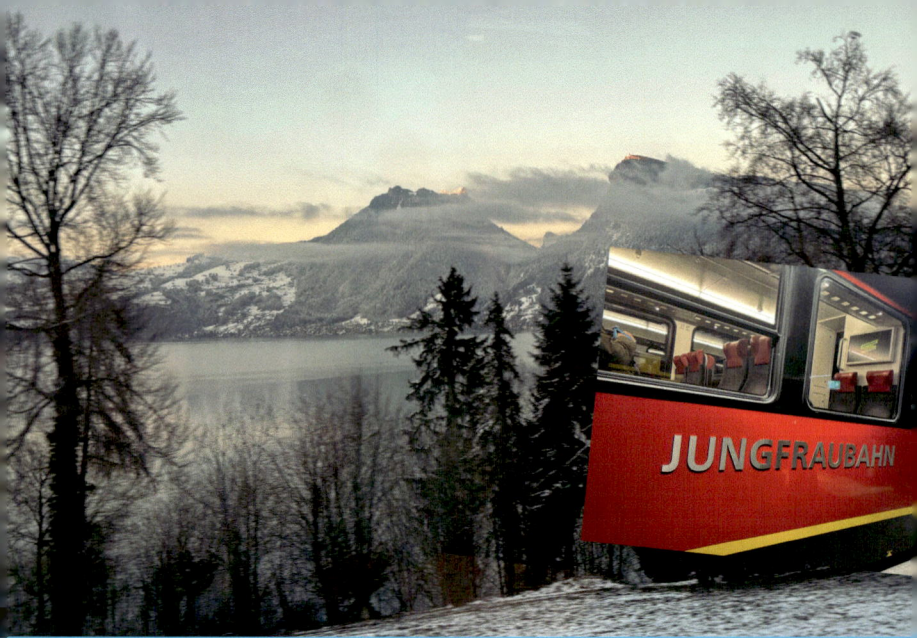

Switzerland: Trains, Snow and Fondue

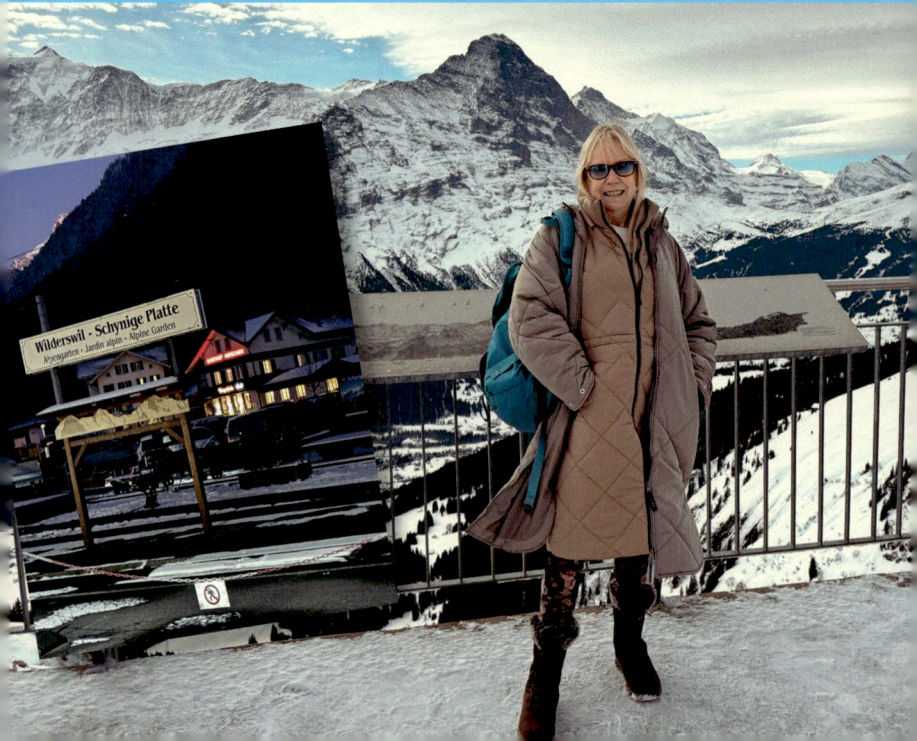

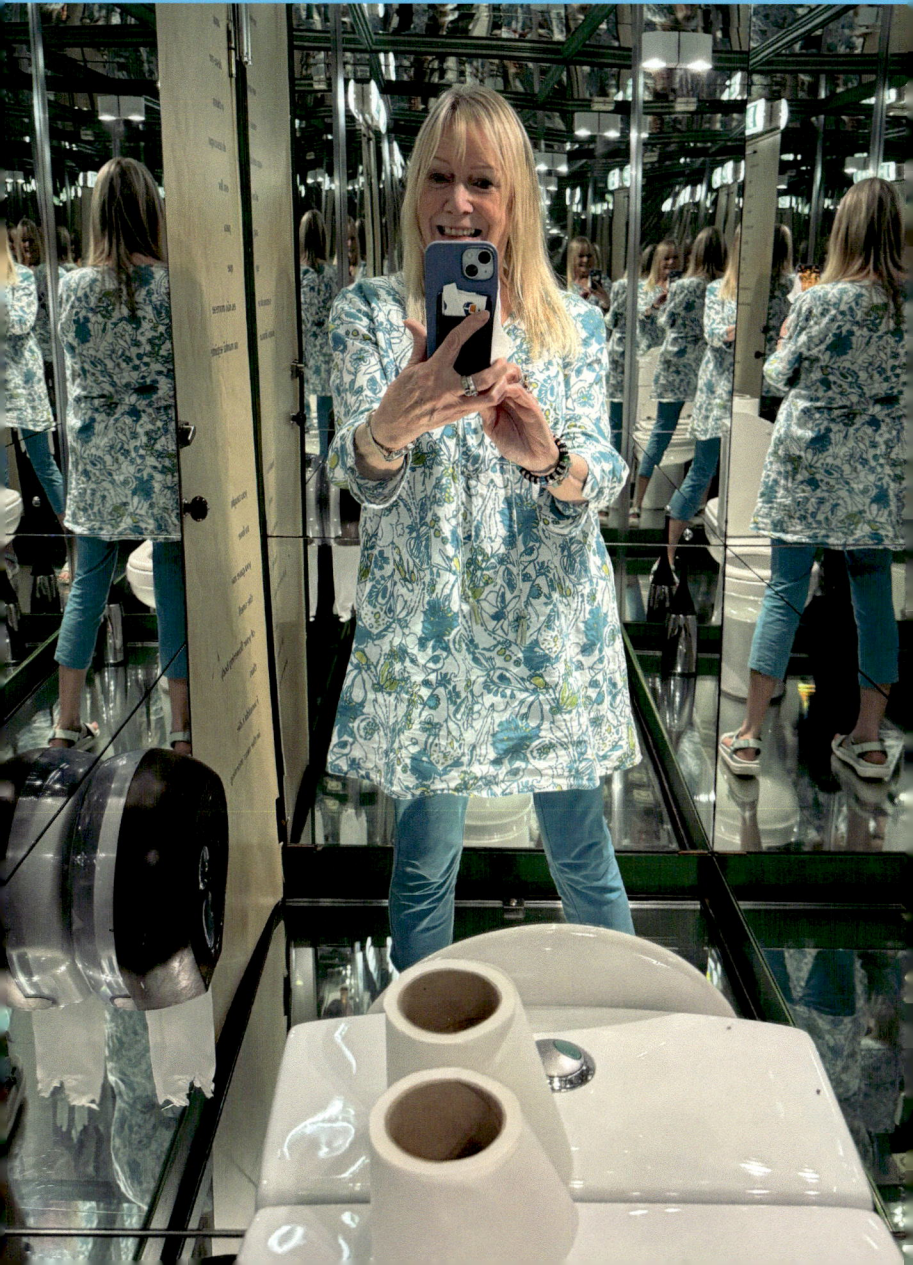

An unforgettable encounter with a toilet in Ecuador

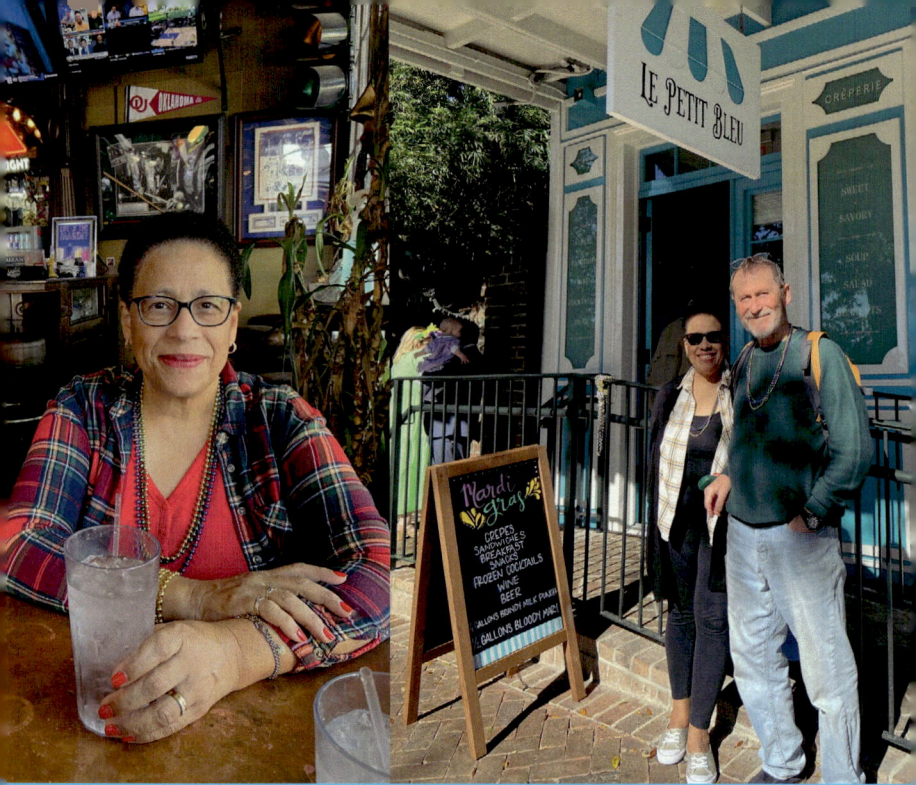

Back to the USA, fifty years on

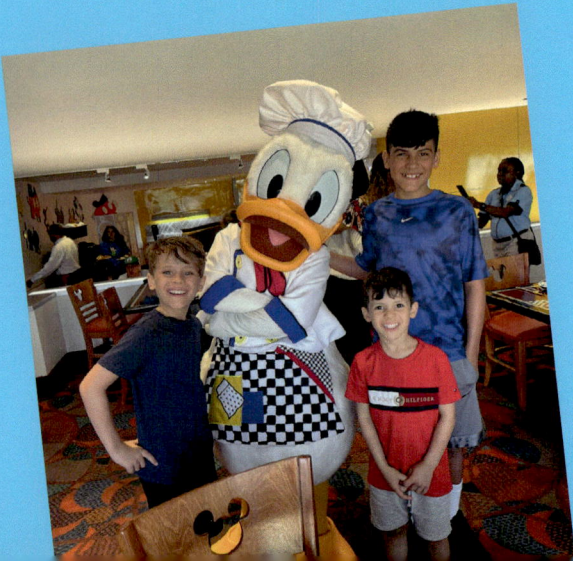

Disney magic!

Thirteen

Switzerland: Travelling with Crohn's *and* a Brain Injury. Trains, Snow and Fondue.

2024

This is a country I had never travelled to before but I knew was a favourite with my parents and sister. Following a head injury which meant I was unable to fly long haul and make a planned trip to Australia and New Zealand, I decided to try something different and take a train journey. I found a company and booked a pretty expensive trip, made even more so by the single supplement. This is always something which annoys me, as I am often a solo traveller. I was anxious about the trip on a few counts. Lifting my suitcase onto trains was one thing that worried me, so I contacted Headway, the brain injury association, and got a brain injury ID card to wear around my neck. This would mean that it would be recognised that I had a valid reason for requesting help. I bought an extra-light suitcase and then proceeded to fill it with so many warm clothes it felt heavy. Knowing nothing about it but being prompted by a friend, I booked some travel assistance. To my surprise and delight, it is free. I was given a booking number and told to present myself at the railway station and all would be fine.

The week before I left, I had a scan of my bowel and was told that it was not looking too bad but as ever there was some inflammation and that wretched piece ten centimetres long, which is severely restricted, was discussed. Nothing new there then but it always serves to remind me of how careful I must be with what I eat. I contacted the rail journey company to explain about my "issues" and explained in particular about my dietary needs. I was assured that all would be fine and I would be able to negotiate. I pondered on what I knew of the national cuisine of Switzerland. Cheese! Fondue! That would be fine, although not so great for cholesterol levels, I guess. Chocolate. All good there except for the nagging pre-diabetic warning I had some time ago, meaning I try to cut down on sugar. Rosti… should be OK as long as there are no skins on the potato. Birchermüesli… hmm, probably too many nuts. As Switzerland is landlocked, I knew fish would not be abundant and I knew it would be heavy on meat, which is mostly a no go. Well, I had managed in so many countries around the world so far that I felt optimistic! I received an email from the tour guide which I finally found in my junk mail outlining the menu for the first day. I emailed him back explaining all of the things which would need slight adjustment and felt hopeful.

Dear Jo,

Further to our chat this pm the Le Dix Menu for Friday evening 19th is:

Starter: Butternut cream soup or Onion Tart and green Salad.

Mains: Beef chuck, beer sauce, alsatian noodles & vegetables or Sea bass, riesling sauce, sauerkraut, potatoes or vegetable tian (zucchinis, eggplants, tomatoes, onions.

Dessert: Panna Cotta with plum compote & hazelnut crumble or Fruit Salad.

If you have any queries about this please let me know.

Kind Regards

C

Hi C,

Sorry, this went into my junk mail. Can't eat beef but can have sea bass but probably not sauerkraut and can't eat eggplant because of the skin. Would need to check whether potatoes have skins. All the rest is fine. Oh actually if plums have skins I can't have those and can't eat nuts. Fruit salad always tricky because of skins but I guess I can just be careful with the compote and just eat the panna cotta. So sorry.

Best wishes

Jo

18ᵗʰ January 2024

I decide to travel the day before the trip starts and stay in London to cut down on the stress in the morning. I present myself for travel assistance and am greeted by a very helpful lady who escorts me to the train with my bag and puts me in the coach near to the refreshments area. I had never noticed before that this is the coach for travellers who need assistance. Also being escorted is a blind woman who sits in the same coach, and I hear them arranging that someone will get her cup of tea en route. On arrival at London Liverpool Street Station, I alight from the coach and there is a wheelchair waiting for me. I explain that this is unnecessary but that I just need a hand with my suitcase. I am escorted to the Underground, where someone helps me, luckily, because there are a lot of steps to navigate. He phones ahead and I am met at the other end by someone who takes my bag and escorts me via a lift to the exit of St Pancras. I cannot be more impressed with the travel assistance service at this point. I have often reflected how difficult it must be for people with physical disabilities to travel on the Underground, as there are often steps and escalators and no lifts. It must make planning every journey quite difficult. The hardest bit of the next part of my journey is just pushing my suitcase on the bumpy pavement. Unscathed, I arrive at the Travelodge.

Day One, Friday

I decide to take a taxi from the Travelodge to St Pancras, as manoeuvring the suitcase on the pavement had been tricky, even with the fancy four-wheeled version. I am charged an extortionate amount for a five-minute journey.

I realise that I have already lost my water bottle, which must have dropped out of the side of my rucksack, and try to source another one, which is extraordinarily difficult, and I end up with an overpriced version from Starbucks. I make my way to the rail journeys office which says it is next to the champagne bar, which is actually a coffee shop. I meet a fellow traveller, and we have coffee together before heading down to the Eurostar check-in, which is surprisingly not crowded. There is an awkward moment when I need to lift my bag to go through security, but a flash of the lanyard helps, and I am given assistance to haul it onto the ramp. In no time at all, we are bound for Paris. One of the group members sits next to me and within a few minutes we discover we come from the same place in the West Midlands and even know some people in common. Time passes quickly as we chat about places we know and people we might know.

We arrive at Gare du Nord and make a quick transfer across to Gare de l'Est to pick up a train to Strasbourg. I am thrilled to be in Paris, albeit briefly, as it has always been a special place for me. The suitcase behaves itself and there are no steps. When we arrive at Strasbourg, the group separates and several people take a lift outside. It is clear that most of the group are of a certain age and there are a couple of people with mobility problems. Fortunately, our hotel is located right across from the station and we trundle across the road and arrive fifteen minutes before dinner is to be served in a restaurant next door.

Everything goes a bit downhill from here, as the restaurant doesn't seem to have been informed of my difficulties with food and there is very little I can eat. I ask for a bowl of salad and am given a small bowl of lettuce and tomatoes. I eat the panna cotta and leave feeling hungry. Note to self: always remember to bring supplies to eat. I have got careless. Sitting on a train seems to have made me extraordinarily, tired so I head for bed.

Day Two, Saturday

Breakfast is fine with lots of choice, and we head off to see a little of the city before catching the next train. We walk to the stunning Cathédrale Notre-Dame-de-Strasbourg at a very slow pace and then I head off with two others to discover Petite-France, with its beautiful cobblestone streets, canals and half-timbered houses. Time for a coffee and I remember that France doesn't seem to sell decaffeinated coffee, so I settle for hot chocolate and a slice of traditional cake. We head back to the hotel to pick up our suitcases to learn that the train has been delayed due to a French rail strike but only for an hour. Eventually we board and we are bound for Basel, then Interlaken and then Wilderswil. As we speed through the countryside, my co-traveller points out the different mountains. She clearly loves this place and has happy memories of being here on holidays with her husband before he died. The sun is setting, and we catch glimpses of it disappearing over the mountain tops. The lakes are tinged red and small villages almost twinkle in the twilight with their snow-topped roofs reflecting off the setting sun. It is truly magical. Train travel is the way to go to get the benefit of this and I am mesmerised, trying to catch photos of the scenery through the window as we speed by. We alight at Wildserwil Station, where there is still a lot of snow on the pavements. After a ten-minute walk, we arrive at a cute-looking hotel, which I learn has a restaurant with a Michelin star. To be investigated further… I think Switzerland has my heart already.

My expectations are about to be dashed. They bring out a cabbage dish with some sauce on, which I had interpreted as noodles. In fact, it definitely said noodles on the menu, and I thought I would be safe with this. The cabbage is very undercooked and apart from not looking very appetising, it seems like a risk. No more food arrives for a while. I speak with the waitress, who is fantastic, as no help is forthcoming from the guide. I write on a piece of paper a list of what I can and can't eat and offer some tentative suggestions. Omelette perhaps? I go to bed hungry…

Day Three, Sunday

The following morning, I am excited to see porridge at breakfast but my first spoonful reveals that it is full of nuts and pomegranate seeds. I can't have that then! I explain my predicament to the long-suffering waitress, and we agree that she will prepare a dish of overnight oats with some soy milk to keep in the fridge just for me all week. She will add some banana. I am very grateful for her thoughtfulness but must admit I wonder what state the banana will be in after a few days. Don't look a gift horse in the mouth, I remind myself.

The highlight of this trip promises to be the experience on the Jungfrau, the "Top of Europe". What is extraordinary is that someone actually had the idea to blast their way through the sheer rock of two mountains, the Eiger and the Mönch, to build a railway right to the summit of the Jungfrau. Many lives were lost during this process. Looking at the map, which we eat our breakfast off, we can see the train lines from Wilderswil to Lauterbrunnen to Kleine Scheidegg and then what looks like a very steep climb up to Jungfraujoch via Eigergletscher.

We set off and after boarding a number of different trains, we finally get on the red one which has *Jungfraubahn* emblazoned across the side. I believe this is the cogwheel train which will take us right to the summit. We are all wearing layers and layers of clothes as rumour has it we will be looking at temperatures of minus twenty-two outside at the top. We finally reach the "Top of Europe" and here we are at the highest accessible point of 3,463 metres. Inside! Feeling extremely overheated, we follow the arrows and finally come out onto a viewing platform. Snowy wonderland is how it is described and that is quite true. A bit grey and no blue sky but clear. It is minus eight and I am not even wearing my hat and gloves. After ten minutes, my fingers turn a bit blue, so we go back inside and head towards the Ice Palace. I have to say that I find this very disappointing. I have a vision in my head, and it is not the one I see in front of me. I am thinking Narnia, ice queen, the White Witch, that sort of thing. A very slippery path leads inside. I try out the Yaktrax and that seems to make the slipperiness even worse, so I just cling onto the rail and make my way extremely slowly forwards. Finally, I arrive in front of some ice sculptures. I think one is a polar bear and the other resembles two dolphins, but surely not. With hindsight, I think they are probably penguins. What is extraordinary, though, is how this was actually built in the 1930s with guides using picks and saws. I am so worried about sliding over that I make my way carefully back to the entrance. I think I may have missed some of it. It's funny how what you visualise in your head isn't exactly how something turns out. I don't like the tourist element, the overpriced fast food, and gift shop selling expensive souvenirs. I do, however, like the Lindt chocolate shop but there are some terrible reviews of this on Tripadvisor, so maybe this is just because I am hungry and like chocolate.

We make our way back to Wilderswil via Kleine Scheidegg and Grindelwald. I love these names. You just want to keep saying them out loud. A lovely day but very overpriced in all. Dinner is a huge disappointment, and I go to bed feeling a bit peckish again.

Day Four, Monday

On Monday, we take a train to Interlaken, which means "between the lakes", which are Lake Thun and Lake Brienz. We walk past Hotel du Lac and ponder on whether this is the hotel Anita Brookner's novel was based on but, in fact, I read that the character in this book sought refuge on the shores of Lake Geneva. It seems that at this time of year a lot of things are closed, and the main focus is on skiing. The proposed boat trip looks as if it won't be happening. The tourist office is open, and they suggest a walk to Neuhaus where there will be a boat which will go around Lake Thun. The footpath around the side of the lake is a bit treacherous-looking, as the snow hasn't yet melted and there is ice in places, but my companion and I take it very slowly. The views of the lake are beautiful, and the sun comes out. Arriving at Neuhaus, we don't have long to wait for a boat and spend an hour and a half drinking tea and looking again at the splendid views of the peaks of the Eiger, the Mönch and the Jungfrau from a different perspective. This is the largest lake in the Bernese Oberland. A bus ride back to Interlaken gives us an opportunity to use our Swiss half-price pass. We manage to get another bus back to Wilderswil where we are looking forward to our fondue night.

This is another food disaster. They are trying so hard to be helpful but it's so complicated to explain the difficulties that Crohn's disease presents for me. No, I can't eat meat, but I am not a vegetarian either, as there are some vegetarian dishes I can't have and skins on vegetables have to be avoided. I opt for the veggie option, however, and they bring me a pot of my own to cook my vegetables in so that they don't touch the meat. Bless them, but they don't get the issue at all. We help ourselves to salad, which is also a bit restricted for me, but I gamely help myself to the bits I can have, missing out the nuts and bean dishes. I am then presented with a dish which contains chopped carrots, broccoli and courgettes and I am meant to cook these in the… water? No cheese in sight. How can you have a fondue without cheese? My fellow travellers are equally disappointed as they cook slices of meat in their devices. Chips arrive. I really want to have a whole bowl to myself, but they are to share. Oh well… More cheese afterwards to fill up! My stomach growls when I head to bed.

Day Five, Tuesday

The next day we catch a train to Grindelwald and decide to get a cable car up to the top of the mountain. The views are spectacular, and I much prefer to be outside with the skiers looking at the views than the ones I had from the inside of a viewing area at the top of the Jungfrau. The intense whiteness of the snow and the beautiful clean air make me gasp with pure pleasure. There is not much to do in Grindelwald apart from shop for ski gear, so along with a couple of my fellow travellers, we decide to take a bus and go up in another cable car to the Männlichen mountain, which is 2,343 metres high. There are superb views in every direction and if you know what you are looking at, you can see Grindelwald, Eiger, Mönch and Jungfrau. I believe that this would be a great place to walk from but not during this season. Intrepid explorer that I am, I have persuaded the others that we should then get another cable car back down to Wengen. That meant traversing a stretch of snow which is mainly meant for skiers. Only people on skis seem to have ventured up here but again the views and the mountain air are just breathtaking and it is all worth it. We take the cable car to Wengen for a hot drink before catching a train back to Wilderswil for some more extraordinary food.

Day 6, Wednesday

A free day on Wednesday sees a few of us heading on the train to Lucerne. This is a two-hour journey but the views through the train windows are fabulous, so it is not a boring trip. I have read about the famous Kapellbrücke (Chapel Bridge) and you can see this as soon as you leave the railway station. This bridge caught fire in 1993 and a lot of the old artwork was destroyed. All that could be saved were two bridgeheads, but it was actually rebuilt over a period of eight months. We explore the Old Town and then visit the Sammlung Rosengart Museum, where a whistle-stop tour takes us around works by Picasso, Klee, Matisse and Kandinsky.

The final night's dinner is very disappointing. I am not given the starter as it contains mushrooms and that is on my can't eat list, but nothing was served in its place. They bring me some soup in a cup which is different from the soup served to others so I can only assume they think it might contain something I can't eat. I haven't managed to explain that if pureed, everything is fine to digest. The main course contains a lump of very tough meat with potatoes. I can only eat the potatoes and ask for a few more. The dessert is covered with nuts and fruit, so they give me scoop of sorbet in its place. Still hungry!

This trip was a challenge for me in more ways than one. The brain injury meant that for the first time I needed travel assistance and had some concerns about my mobility and lifting luggage, not to mention potentially slipping over on ice. Wearing a lanyard was an asset and I found fellow travellers to be helpful. Anglia Rail was extraordinary with their assistance. Travel For London turned out to be not as reliable and a bit hit and miss. On the return journey on the Underground, I found someone to ask for help, but he assured me that no one would help pick up my case in case they hurt their back. He said that he was a union representative and called forwards to Liverpool Street Station but then informed me I could get no help. It seems that some staff are more helpful than others, which is not great for travellers with a major physical disability. I need to investigate this further.

Switzerland is famous for its scenic rail journeys and winter sports. It is also renowned for its "delectable cuisine" but sadly I did not really get to enjoy this. It is expensive too. I would love to visit in the summer where I guess the beauty of nature would be different but equally enthralling.

The learning experience for me was being able, in a very small way, to step into the shoes of someone who may find the mechanics of travel a barrier. With regard to the culinary experience, I realise that all-inclusive in the form of meals is not the way to go for me and something I have experienced very little of in my travels. I think I will dig out the old fondue set and invite a few people round for dinner!

Postscript

I contacted the company with my concerns, and they were extremely apologetic and gave me a voucher for £200 off one of their trips. I am planning my next trip and will phone ahead myself to discuss my dietary requirements with the hotel.

I was recently discharged from the hospital and here is a sentence included in the letter from the consultant neurosurgeon: "I have advised Joanna that she can return to her normal activities including riding horses, flying and 'race across the world' if her application is successful." We'll see…

Fourteen

An Unforgettable Encounter with a Toilet in Ecuador

2010

I have had some extraordinary moments in toilets, some of which are described in this book. The most recent peculiar experience was this year when I went to a toilet in a restaurant in Madeira. It was full of mirrors, up above, by your side and underneath. It was fascinating and I just had to take a photo... but I digress... I can't complete this book without reference to something that happened to me involving a toilet in Ecuador.

Saturday, 14ᵗʰ August 2010

I am in Quito, Ecuador where I have just finished a stint of volunteering. I have been working at a place called the Extreme Response Centre in Zámbiza, which is located next to the city dump. Quito's poorest residents work here, and I have been working looking after their children in the Day Care Centre on the site. I have come along with a friend from the UK to work here as a volunteer for a few weeks.

We are staying with a family in the new part of town, and they have gone away for the weekend. We are planning to leave on a bus to go to Lima on Monday night but have a weekend to relax after volunteering. The family have kindly agreed that we can stay until then. I wake up and as usual I need the toilet straight away, so I head to the bathroom. I pull the chain, and it doesn't work. I try again. Still nothing, so I decide to investigate by lifting the top off the cistern. It slips from my hand and falls somehow into the toilet and that is when the water starts to gush out. I have no idea what to do! I look around for a way of stopping the water. I shout for my friend, who is in his room in a different part of the house. Eventually, he arrives at the door, looking sleepy, and surveys the scene. I am yelling at him, and I am wearing a very skimpy nightie. It is awkward. He looks nonplussed. We can't work out how to stem the flow of water and we are beginning to paddle in it.

"Quick," I yell. "Grab those towels."

The family's bathrobes are on the back of the door, along with their towels. We grab them all and try to mop up the water. It's not working.

I decide to run for help and dash out through the front door shouting, "*Necesitas ayuda!*"

It is not the best area to be outside in your nightie, but a man comes to help. I gesture that he must come with me inside the house. He looks worried but I am being very insistent, so he follows me. We dash to the bathroom, and he surveys the scene. He nods sagely, leans down and turns off the stopcock. The water stops. He leaves. My friend and I breathe a sigh of relief and look at the devastation I have caused. The water is beginning to move into the hallway outside the bathroom.

"Keep wiping it up," I shout. "I'll look for mops!"

I pull on some clothes on top of my nightie and go back into the street and head for the little shop at the end of the road. I look for mops, buckets and cloths and try to explain to the shopkeeper what I am looking for in my limited Spanish, throwing in a bit of role play to help her to imagine the scene. My friends know that I do this when I can't think of the words I need in a different language. It usually works. I am doing a mopping movement on the floor to show her what I mean but as I stand up, I bang the side of my face on a shelf somehow, which results in a nosebleed. Can this get any worse? She has no mops or buckets but hands me some cloths and tissues for my bleeding nose.

I head back to the house, and we continue with the mop-up operation. My friend doesn't ask me about my bloody nose. I think he has had enough of me so far today. We hang the sodden bathrobes and towels over the side of the small balcony, hoping they will dry off so we can hang them back on the door before the family return. I wonder whether they have insurance to cover the toilet, but I have a feeling things don't work that way here.

The next day, the towels have dried out! The family return later and don't seem too worried about the toilet.

Luckily, there is another one in the house. Martha (the mother) says she will call the *fontanero* (plumber) in the morning.

Monday, 16th August

The *fontanero* arrives and I surreptitiously listen in to the conversation. Martha appears to be choosing colours for a whole new bathroom suite. Yes, I was right, they don't have household insurance, but she is expecting me to pay. I try to explain about insurance and hope that the company I volunteered with may foot the bill, but I do explain it probably won't be for the whole bathroom. My friend and I while the hours away until it is time to leave for the bus station. I think the family are quite glad to wave us goodbye. We didn't mention the bathrobes.

Postscript

I had to pay for the toilet. The company didn't stretch to that, and I don't think that they had experienced such a claim before. I have never again lifted the lid on a cistern but then again, they aren't built like that any longer, fortunately!

Fifteen

Maud Returns to America - Fifty Years On!

2024

This chapter was written by a very good friend, "Maud".

Background – September 2019

I'm returning home from a conference in London and it's late. As I enter the house and without much warning, I'm vomiting over the toilet pan in serious pain. Sweat is dripping off my body. I'm on the floor, naked and finding it hard to breathe. Fear grips me and I'm thinking, *am I dying?*

Now it's February 2020 and I'm in a supermarket toilet in France. It's happening again. It's early afternoon, my husband and two young grandsons are with me, I haven't eaten much today – except for a meal replacement drink. Vomiting, gripping onto the handrail in the toilet, terrible stomach pain under my ribs, sweat pouring off me.

Oh my God now I am *dying – and in a toilet!*

No, *clearly* I didn't die! Back from our holiday, I'd made a doctor's appointment and whilst getting dressed from a scan which had swiftly followed, she tells me that it looks like I have gallstones.

That's not so bad, I'm thinking, *just means I need to manage my diet better, perhaps lose a bit of weight.* A few minor episodes follow over the next few months, then, during another violent and very painful event, I tell my husband I have to go to A and E.

What follows has been life-changing.

It's September 2020. Covid-19 is in full swing and at the end of a week's hospital stay (during which no one could have any visitors), I'm told I have pancreatic cancer. Weeks of scans and tests follow. I'm very scared because I'm actually not prepared for dying – yet. We run an early years setting employing ten people, I have four young grandchildren, not to mention a husband, and three grown-up children, a brother and three sisters. We are a close family. How do I prepare for dying? With massive support from family, close friends and work colleagues, I somehow manage to stay quite calm – and remember to breathe.

It's 17th November (just over two months and two cancellations from my diagnosis) and I'm about to undergo a nine-hour operation to remove two-thirds of my pancreas, my spleen and gallbladder. If successful, any potentially cancerous tumours will be removed – but I might develop Type 1 diabetes. Well, it would actually be Type 3c diabetes, because I'll only have a partial pancreas left, so will, in all likelihood, not produce sufficient insulin.

I will have to take antibiotics and pancreatic enzyme replacement therapy (PERT) for the rest of my life. As I recover over the next few weeks, I'm told that, thankfully, I don't have to undergo chemotherapy.

February 2021, and a blood test reveals that I have indeed developed diabetes and will be prescribed metformin tablets. Eighteen months later and I'm prescribed insulin (Humulin I). Although I knew this might happen, I'm actually very upset because it seems that my body is out of control.

January 2023. I get the news that tumours have developed in the remaining third of my pancreas – and that I need to undergo a "total pancreatectomy".

27th February 2023, and I can feel the icy-cold anaesthetic creeping up my hand. If I'm "lucky", by the time I wake up, portions of my small intestine and stomach, bile duct and remaining pancreas will have been removed. The alternative is too grim to entertain, so I decide not to go there. Either way, I'll spend my seventieth birthday (March 2023) in hospital. Some might say that by seventy I've had a good innings, but I don't look or feel my age… and I've got lots of living yet to do!

Fast forward to January 2024. Without the following medication, my life expectancy is limited:

* I wear a Libre 2 sensor on my arm, which has to be replaced on alternate arms every two weeks. The sensor monitors my glucose levels and is a lifesaver. An alarm goes off on my mobile phone if my glucose level dips below four or goes above twenty. My "reading" should be between four and ten;

* I currently inject twelve units of Lantus every morning. This is a long-acting insulin, lowering blood sugar levels, although the number of daily units could change depending on my readings;
* I inject varying units of Fiasp several times throughout every day. The actual number of units for each injection depends on the reading indicated by the sensor;
* I take Creon tablets with every snack or meal (to enable nutrients from the food I eat to be absorbed by my body);
* I take penicillin V (necessary to boost my immune system as a result of having my spleen removed) and omeprazole (to aid the absorption of the Creon) twice a day;
* I take one atorvastatin daily (to reduce my increased risk of stroke and/or heart attack);
* I take Adcal tablets (vitamin D and calcium) twice a day;
* I take Forceval tablets (vitamins and minerals) daily after breakfast;
* I take 1x300mg tablet of ferrous gluconate (iron) daily (should be 2x300mg, but the side effects are still unpleasant);
* I take one each of bisoprolol and amlodipine daily (for high blood pressure);
* I take regular paracetamol and codeine (for back and knee pain);
* I also carry a bag of Jelly Babies – for when my blood sugar (glucose) dips too low.

There is a good reason for that list above, because although I am a frequent (ferry) traveller between the UK and France (where, surprisingly perhaps, no one has ever checked my boxes of medication), holidays further afield have been put on hold. However, by January 2024, it seems reasonable to book the long-planned trip to America – which should have been a celebration of my seventieth birthday the year before. Now it will be a celebration of fifty years since I was last in the US (spending my twenty-first birthday there whilst on a university student exchange to Eastern Michigan University, in Ypsilanti). During that spring term, I'd travelled to New Orleans, New York and across to California and Tijuana on the Mexican border, spending days on the iconic Greyhound buses. For over forty years, I'd bored my husband with my "American tales" and now we were going to experience it together.

Preparations – January 2024

So, having obtained an ESTA for entry to the US and travel insurance sufficient to cover existing medical conditions, I start looking at flights. The first hurdle is refrigeration: insulin needs to be refrigerated. No airlines will provide a refrigeration service, and I can understand why. I decide that an insulated lunch bag with frozen icepacks seems the answer for my eight-hour flight. I also need to book hotels that offer an in-room fridge – which several add a top-up charge for.

Next, I need to work out the amount of medication I will need to take with me, to last the four weeks we'd be away (enough to fill a small suitcase, as it happened).

I spend hours researching what paperwork I need to provide in order to get through airport security, and what evidence I could provide to support the fact that I have a "hidden disability". Apart from the implications of my glucose levels going either too high or too low and therefore having to eat at regular intervals (including taking supplies of food in case of delays), I frequently and urgently need to use the toilet. This isn't due to the diabetes, per se, but to the side effects of the medication and the fact that food can go through my system very quickly.

Strangely, it's always very late at night that my brain goes into overdrive, so that I'm frequently still awake at 2 or 3am! That's why, in the early hours of this January morning, I happen to successfully apply for a National Disability Card (for myself) and a Carers Card (for my husband). I also apply for two accessible toilet keys. I already had a bracelet that said "Type 1 Diabetes", but growing anxiety leads me to order a second one: this one says "Diabetes on Insulin".

I contact my doctor's surgery, as my late-night research makes it clear that I need a doctor's letter to explain the reason for the medication. I also print off a Medical Device Awareness Card (explaining why I shouldn't pass through some full-body scanners or X-ray machines with my diabetes sensor, as they can damage the device). I also print off the copy for airport personnel. According to the advice, when going through security, I could request a "pat-down", instead.

There's a lot of very useful advice online about travelling with Type 1 diabetes, but, bizarrely, the more I read and the more I try to remember what I need to pack, the more stressed I start to feel. Have I prepared well enough? Do I have everything I need? This isn't helped by the fact that, arriving at my doctor's surgery (at the allotted time) to collect my letter, I'm told that they no longer write letters – just list all the prescribed medication. Well! To be honest, that's not particularly helpful, as much of it reads like gobbledegook to the untrained medical eye.

Arriving at the Airport – February 2024

When booking our tickets, I had decided to tick the box that said "request assistance", as the airport blurb had indicated that there was likely to be a long walk from check-in to our flight gate. Still, I'm quite surprised that a wheelchair and a Hidden Disabilities Sunflower lanyard are readily available shortly after checking in our suitcases. My husband pulls our two carry-on cases and carries his rucksack on his back, while I have my "lunch bag" on my lap with enough insulin pens for four weeks, two spare Libre 2 sensors, immediate medication, a packet of biscuits, a small yoghurt and two icepacks, along with my handbag and a plastic wallet containing all the necessary paperwork. A quiet but very helpful lady pushes me in my wheelchair, which I actually find a bit embarrassing. However, it *was* a long way from check-in to security and it *was* very busy with long queues, but with her help we're able to use the priority lanes.

Then we arrive at airport security and my nightmare begins.

A very loud, harassed lady approaches my quiet lady demanding to know what was going on and asks her who I am – she doesn't actually speak to me. She acts as if I am invisible. After explaining, Loud Lady brusquely tells Quiet Lady that she can go and then turns to me, saying I need to put everything on the conveyer belt. I start to get out my paperwork to show her (including the Medical Device Awareness Card), but she's already shouting into her walkie-talkie to someone and walks across to another belt.

A different person says, "You need to put everything onto the conveyer belt and empty out that lunch bag."

With that, she starts to open my small carry-on case, which contains the spare medication, toiletries (all less than 10ml) and a change of underwear. She looks a bit surprised and asks what the medication is, so I hand *her* my paperwork. She scrutinises it but keeps shaking her head. Whilst I'm talking to her, trying to explain, she shouts across to Loud Lady to come and see what I've given her. I actually feel like a criminal.

It's hard to describe the noise and the total chaos that's going on around me. My husband is ushered through a different security check, even though he's saying he's with me and needs to wait. At that point, and for some reason, I start to cry – and Loud Lady is clearly exasperated.

With each of us on either side of the barrier, I'm eventually given a "pat down" by a much calmer person who explains what the procedure entails, where she would put her hands, and asks if I want to go somewhere private.

I reply, "No, but I need my bags."

By this time, my lunch bag is being opened and each

item taken out – including the icepacks, which are being scrutinised and about to be thrown away. Literally held above a bin!

I shout out, "You cannot throw them away. I need them for my insulin!"

She stops, looks at me as if I'm mad and puts them back in the bag having passed her Taser gun over them. Then she says that the yoghurt will have to go. To save space, I'd discarded the outer cardboard. She aggressively tells me that the yoghurt pot itself doesn't show how much is in it. It's 75ml, but she's having none of it.

I look across to see where my husband is and see that he's trying to gather together our belongings which have been spread into several different trays. My handbag, our passports and the plastic wallet with all my paperwork are nowhere to be seen. At this point, a woman who'd been looking at me during this whole fiasco approaches and hugs me… which makes me start crying all over again.

This isn't the way I'd envisaged our holiday starting and I know this is why I'm so upset. I'm also very angry, and hot, but I know that making a scene isn't going to help.

Of course, eventually everything is found. We repack our cases and can begin to relax once we get to the departure lounge – and find a loo.

America
First Stop, New Orleans, Louisiana

Hours later, after a long and uncomfortable flight, we arrive at Louis Armstrong International Airport. We're tired but excited. The wait to get through Homeland Security is calm and quiet – but interminable! So, of course, our pre-booked taxi won't wait unless we pay double the price. Determined not to be fazed, we agree to pay and eventually exit into the cool New Orleans night air. Unfortunately for me, I now desperately need the toilet, which I know is just back into the airport entrance. I haven't previously mentioned how quickly this can come on, but suffice to say, it's the reason I carry spare clothing, wet wipes and a plastic bag. By the time I'm back outside, the taxi is about to be moved on by airport security and I'm wondering what exactly I did wrong in a previous life!

Eventually, we get to our hotel. It's Mardi Gras season and New Orleans is *alive!* All past annoyances are forgotten, and we head out in search of food. Every day we walk for miles around the city, following the floats and screaming for the beads and trinkets being thrown out into the crowds. It's exhilarating. We talk and laugh with total strangers, buy light-up hats, eat po' boys and oysters (the first time for me) and drink cocktails, adjusting my insulin injections according to my sensor readings. Of course, we always manage to wangle toilet keys, even though all the bars and hotels have signs that say the "Restrooms are for Customers Only".

Next Stop, New York... and It Is Freezing!

After an amazing week, it's time for our flight to New York – where, unfortunately, my suitcase doesn't turn up on baggage reclaim. A good reason for packing essentials into your hand luggage. But as a result of one of my late-night forays on the internet, I'd taken a photograph of our cases before we checked in at Heathrow. This is just as well, as the airline are able to locate it and deliver it to our hotel two days later.

During our four days in New York, we visit Ground Zero, the John Lennon memorial in Central Park, the Empire State Building, and other notable locations. Wearing the Sunflower lanyard given to me at the airport is interesting. The guides at the Empire State Building have clearly been given training and usher me through the fast lanes without me asking. Also, the same thing happens at LaGuardia Airport as we leave for our next stop (Detroit).

A word of caution if, like me, urgent access to a toilet is crucial. Most buses do not have toilets! So, halfway through our "Hop On, Hop Off" bus tour of the city, I feel the tell-tale signs. Within minutes, it's desperate – can't even risk getting off to go looking for a toilet. Luckily, we're almost at our hotel stop, but not in time to prevent an accident. We get off and I walk very uncomfortably through the lobby to the lift and up to our room. Not good. But after a bath, a change of clothes and two codeine tablets (side effect, constipation), we're off out walking down to the Hudson River and Wall Street.

Detroit, San Francisco, Los Angeles, San Diego... and Back to New Orleans

Apart from finding my old halls of residence (Sellars) at EMU, which was amazingly nostalgic, the place I most wanted to visit was "Hitsville" – the Motown Museum. It can't have been there back in '74, and if it was, it definitely wasn't on our tour list back then. We were due to fly out to San Francisco later in the day, so I'd booked a slot for late morning. The sound of Motown was the backdrop to our lives during our teens and twenties and my husband is a real music buff. So, standing in the very studio where the songs were recorded, hearing about Berry Gordy and how those Motown stars were groomed for stardom (in the true sense of the word) was like experiencing history.

Our four-week holiday in the US was amazing. Apart from a few night-time hypos (which necessitated getting through my stash of Jelly Babies), I was careful to plan journeys around medication and toilet needs. Although not ideal, codeine became my best friend as there was never such a thing as a rest day. The Golden Gate Bridge, Sausalito, Alcatraz, Haight Ashbury, Alamo Square and the Painted Ladies, Fisherman's Wharf and Celebrating Chinese New Year in San Francisco: these were not to be missed. Although I had wanted to capture that experience of fifty years ago by travelling via Greyhound, booking a hire car proved to be a great idea. We could stop whenever I needed to – and we often did.

One of my sons is a real "tree-hugger" and was over the moon when we visited the Sequoia National Park en route to LA. "Park" is definitely a misnomer: it's a huge wilderness! Whilst there are no cafés (possibly so as not to invite bears!), there were at least several public toilets.

The Getty Museums in LA and Malibu were a highlight, as was the Warner Bros studio tour, Muscle Beach (Santa Monica), finding Rodeo Drive and the Beverley Wilshire hotel from *Pretty Woman*. We'd booked a lovely modern hotel in an area just outside LA called Calabasas in the Malibu Canyons and we played Joni Mitchell's "Ladies of the Canyon" on the car radio. On our way back from San Diego, we stopped off at La Jolla Cove to see the hundreds of seals and sea lions lazing on the rocks. Magical!

When we returned to New Orleans for the last few days of our stay, we booked several trips we hadn't had time for during Mardi Gras: cemetery tours (including the tomb of Marie Laveau – the witch queen of New Orleans) and river tours through the Bayou, where we saw alligators and raccoons in their natural habitat. An interesting fact is that, several years ago, they used to throw marshmallows to the alligators to attract them to the boats, until they discovered that the alligators were getting diabetes. Now they throw protein pellets.

Epilogue

In December 2023, we sold the business we'd owned and run successfully for thirty-three years. So, our America trip in February and March 2024, which was the holiday of a lifetime, also feels like a reward for all those years of hard work and accountability. Not only a birthday celebration and a nostalgic step back in time, but also a triumph over a devasting diagnosis. We had an incredible time.

Thankfully, throughout four internal flights, whilst I still had to show my paperwork and explain why I didn't want to go through the full-body scanners or X-ray machines, there was never once a repeat of what I can only describe as ignorant behaviour on the part of some staff at the airport.

However, I still feel traumatised by that experience, and it has taught me a lot about travelling with a disability:

* I hope I'll be more sympathetic to others who need "assistance", whether the reason is obvious or "hidden";
* I won't let other people intimidate me;
* I'll get a letter from my doctor next time – not a list of my medications;
* Although I didn't need to use it on this occasion, I'll always have adequate travel insurance, should I need medical treatment abroad;
* I'll ensure I take sufficient medication, toiletries and a change of clothes *in my carry-on case*;
* I'll always carry spare clothes and wet wipes (for times I'm taken short!).

The most important thing, though, is that I will be travelling again soon!

Sixteen

Visiting Florida with Neurodivergent Children

2024

This chapter was written by Maud's son-in-law.

My wife and I are planning a holiday to America with our three sons. Our eldest is twelve, our middle child is eight and has a diagnosis of autism and ADHD, and our youngest is five, with a diagnosis of ADHD and is on the autism pathway. We are planning to go on a two-week holiday to Florida to visit the theme parks. The boys' neurodivergence can mean they struggle to wait, queue or sit/stand still. They can often struggle with following direction and may choose to refuse to do something or just walk off and do something else, which can make travel or waiting in lines and queues highly challenging, as you can imagine.

We make the decision not to tell our children too far in advance, as they may struggle to contain their excitement and become dysregulated at school. We tell them three days before we leave. They are very excited and struggle a little. One complains that we shouldn't have told them so early as he is too excited! They manage well, however.

Two months before the holiday, I begin contacting the relevant companies to procure support during our holiday. I contact the airport's Special Assistance Team, informing them of our travel dates and the needs of our party. A few days later, I speak to a member of the team on the phone for about an hour. They are lovely and very keen to help. Whilst they cannot guarantee certain queue-skipping, they arrange a Special Assistance Pass Card that we can show to any team member, and we are assured that they will help us in whatever way they can. They give us details of the sensory room at the airport, should we need it during our time waiting for our flight. They give me details of how to contact the Transportation Security Administration (TSA) to alert them of our return flight and book the children in with a service which provides a representative to support you through customs and security. They also provide me with a TSA Cares Card for the children to display in the airport, which appears to serve a similar function to the Special Assistance Pass. The representative also places us on a reserve list for bulkhead seats, free of charge, to provide the children with extra space to get up and move around should we need it. We will find out if we will get these seats at check-in. It is also suggested that we could obtain Hidden Disabilities Sunflower lanyards, which the children already have. This is a badge that alerts others quickly that the user has a hidden disability. The representative is very keen to ensure we don't need anything else. She asks and goes through a list of any other adaptations we may need, such as ensuring we don't want to book on any extra baggage items and making sure everyone has the correct meal choice booked. At the end of the call, the lady emails me all the details of everything discussed with all the links to the relevant sites and documents. I am very impressed.

At the airport, the boys are wearing their Sunflower lanyards, and we show the Special Assistance Card. We are directed straight to a check-in desk to avoid the queue and check in efficiently. As we approach airport security, they see our Sunflower lanyards and direct us to a much shorter disabilities lane. We busy the children with trips to shops and games and electrical devices to pass the waiting time and they cope well. At boarding, we are allowed to do so at any time we like, due to our card. We choose to wait for a while so that we don't have to sit too long on the plane waiting for take-off.

As we board, we request that our buggy should arrive when we land so we can put our son in it to assist us immediately and we are told that this will happen. When we sit down in our seats, the head cabin steward approaches and asks if the children will need any extra support on the plane. We tell her that they won't but request if it is possible for them to leave first from the plane (we are next to the door), so the children don't become dysregulated, and we are told this will be fine.

When it is time to disembark, the cabin crew

unload First Class passengers first and the children start becoming dysregulated. The opposite side of the plane is then unloaded. I remind the crew of the arrangement, and they agree we can leave. Unfortunately, there is an error, and the buggy is not available upon disembarking, but we are told it will be dropped to baggage collection shortly.

The boys really struggle with the queue for customs. When we contacted TSA, they were specific that there would be no adaptations for this queue, so we were prepared for this. There is a lot of screaming and crying and we try to contain them and finally we make it through. Unfortunately, the buggy does not arrive and ends up being the final item off the aeroplane. We have to wait an excessive amount of time, and we are the last people who disembarked from the plane still waiting at the baggage claim, which causes the children to become highly dysregulated.

The next day, we are ready to explore! The theme park advertises that you have to book an online meeting thirty days prior to arrival and an interview to receive special support for the park but I seem unable to make this work. Eventually, I ring their US number to ask for advice and I am informed that the online meeting system does not work and that we will need to go to Guest Services in the park and they will decide whether we meet the requirements for support. I offer to bring doctors' letters and our blue badges, but I am informed that they believe that to be intrusive and they just take everybody's needs on merit. When we arrive at our first park, we go to Guest Services and wait for around thirty minutes in the queue where we are offered a Disability Access Pass (DAS). This allows you to join the wait for a ride "virtually" and do things around the park, returning when the wait is complete. You then join the Lightning Line to get onto the ride more quickly. The lady informs us we will not necessarily get a DAS pass but within moments of the meeting, one of the children is climbing a bookshelf and the other is hiding under a desk, so she quickly issues the pass without further ado.

The DAS system of virtually queuing for our rides works quite well. We are able to keep the boys busy and entertained while we queue virtually. It becomes clear, though, that these Lightning Passes can also be purchased by park goers who wish to skip queues, as well as those with disabilities, so the wait was not exactly "lightning fast"! Sometimes these lines seem to be longer than the ordinary lines, which makes it all a bit pointless (a bit like priority boarding at airports now, which are often longer than the other line). We often end up struggling with excessive wait times in these lines, which appears to be through over-selling of the passes, and in effect eradicating the purpose of the DAS support.

As a child, I have fond memories of going to Florida, walking the parks and seeing characters everywhere. I remember leaving the park with a book full of autographs, pictures and happy memories. The big difference today is that there are very few characters walking around, and those that are present are heavily gatekept by miserable staff. We see Chewbacca and the children are extremely excited. They run over but there is a big group of people surrounding him. I try to convince the children to go in and stand next to him for a photo, but they are overwhelmed by so many people. Every time they pluck up the courage and get close, another adult pushes in front of them, making them retreat. I make repeated eye contact with the attendant, pointing at the boys and their hidden disability badges. Eventually, the boys get in to have a photo and the lady immediately drags Chewbacca out of the way and says he is returning backstage. I explain the situation and she aggressively tells me that he won't meet the children, but if they want to see him, they can wait by a nearby plant pot (in the direct sunlight), and he will return shortly. The boys are very disheartened, but we wait to see him. He returns shortly and upsettingly the same scene unfolds. The boys are nervous around all the people that swarm around Chewbacca and they are unable to get close. I make repeated eye contact with the lady, pointing out the badges again, but nothing happens, and she announces that Chewbacca is leaving relatively quickly. I approach her and explain their need, the hidden disability badge, the DAS pass and she says it doesn't matter as they are leaving. She again says that we can wait at the plant pot, and she will make sure that they see him next time. I point out that she had said that previously and it didn't happen, and she gets angry and tells me I can wait or leave and storms off with the character. The boys are devastated.

Unfortunately, this is how every possible character interaction unfolds. There is always an attendant hollering that they can't stop and won't pose for photos and the boys find this very unsettling and upsetting. When we see Kylo Ren from *Star Wars*, the boys are so excited, but they now know that if they don't get really close to him, they won't get to see him. They charge in, get next to him, and he poses for a photo. As I go to take it, the attendant blocks the photo with her body and shouts that we cannot have a photo as the children haven't asked Kylo. Kylo then walks off. The children follow him and politely ask for a photo, but he ignores them. Eventually, the attendant explains that they must be selected at random by Kylo for a photo. This is difficult enough for any child to understand, let alone ones with the needs our children have. As the children are desperate, we actually follow Kylo for around twenty minutes with the children wearing their hidden disability badges. We position ourselves to be a few steps ahead on Kylo's route constantly. He repeatedly ignores them, posing for photos with pretty much everyone except them. At one stage, in a big wide area, he walks up to them and looks at them and they smile and ask for a photo, thinking that finally their time has come! He makes a gesture for them to move out of the way and the attendant shouts at them to move. We leave. On our last trip to a park, we see a character and I ask the children if we should make one last attempt, and they say they don't want to as they are never very nice to them. I tell them otherwise, but frankly, I have to agree.

Universal Studios take a slightly different approach. Prior to our visit, we had to apply for an IBCCES Card. This requires an online application which needs a photo, details of their disability and a piece of evidence from a professional. I had completed this and I was informed that someone would contact me a few days before the trip to clarify and confirm. Luckily, a few days before the trip, the children's cards update from pending to complete. When we arrive at Universal Studios, we have to go Guest Services, much as we did at the other park, to obtain our pass. Universal employ an Attraction Access Pass (AAP). This is more "old-school" and is a physical piece of card that has a table on it for ride names and times. If a ride has less than a twenty-minute wait, you can instantly join the Express Lane. If a ride has more than a twenty-minute wait, the ride attendant will write down a time to return.

There is a downside to this system in that you have to be at the ride to have your return time marked. This means that my wife ends up taking the children to something to keep them busy, while I sprint to the other end of the park, get them to write a wait time on, then sprint back to the children at the other end of the park. On the plus side, we can use the rides which have a shorter wait whilst we are waiting for a long ride. Staff seemed to be using their initiative. They often look at the Express Lane and if it is short, they let us immediately join, sometimes even if the wait is twenty-five or thirty minutes. The biggest difference we also note in comparison with the other park, and are extremely grateful for, is the general manner of the staff at Universal. They all seem brighter and happier. When there is an issue waiting to see Captain America and someone goes in front of the children, the attendant immediately picks up on it. She apologises and talks to the boys while they wait to go next. All of the characters, their attendants and ride staff all seem genuinely happy to see the children and take their time to make them feel special and go that extra mile. I breathe a sigh of relief! I recall the experience yesterday when our cards were scanned and by mistake the staff member deleted something we had waited over an hour for and refused to help and told us to join the queue again. When something similar happens at Universal and an attendant crosses out our wait on the pass card in error, we go to the ride and they apologise profusely, chat and laugh with the children and let us straight on the ride.

Our holiday nears the end. We prepare to return to the UK with some trepidation about how the flight arrangements will unfold. We arrive at Orlando International Airport and, thankfully, when the representative sees our Special Assistance Card, they direct us immediately to priority boarding, which is very helpful. There is, however, some confusion about how to find our TSA Cares representative. We end up in a queue and when we get to the front, the member of staff is quite short with us and annoyed that we are in the wrong place. They radio for a TSA Cares member of staff, who shortly joins us. He is lovely and walks us over to our own little security area and talks with the adults and children throughout to make everyone feel settled. They interject on several occasions to tell the security staff that the children don't need to show their passports, just their boarding cards, and they don't need to remove their shoes, and we can keep our water, but he can just test it. He gets us through security really quickly and we feel very supported. He checks that we are OK and asks if we want him to come through the airport with us and support further, which we decline.

On the monorail to the gate, we spot our cabin crew, who are very sweet and talk to the children. At the gate, we ask a staff cabin steward about our buggy and explain what happened on the flight here. They explain that unfortunately they cannot make a definite promise and are unsure why it was made last time. Due to the size of the buggy, it must go in the hold. The steward states that she can't promise when it will come out, but she really hopes it will appear quickly, and she apologises profusely for what happened last time. On the flight, no representative comes to check if we need anything as they did on the first flight, but all goes smoothly. When it is time to disembark, the staff member notes our Sunflower lanyards and asks if we want to leave with the First Class passengers. She also wishes us luck with our buggy.

When we reach security at Heathrow, we are directed through a disability lane and seen instantly. The customs representative is very patient with the boys, who are now rather irritable after the flight. Thankfully, as this airline has allowed us priority check-in, our bags are first off and, thankfully this time, the buggy appears shortly afterwards. We breathe a sigh of relief.

Despite some of the difficulties and setbacks, we had a fantastic holiday in Orlando. Services were available to support the children and make the visit that little bit easier. Some of them required planning ahead and contacting services in advance and filling in forms. It meant that we travelled with a dossier full of forms, information, passes and lanyards but it was worth it for the support that it provided. On the whole, I felt staff across some of the services appeared to be understanding in supporting our children and their needs. I did feel that there is some room for improvement, perhaps in terms of staff training and in some cases a more helpful attitude, but overall, it feels as if it is moving in the right direction and for that we are very grateful. We look forward to our next trip!

Help Page and Information

The following websites contain information to help those travelling with disabilities, hidden disabilities, chronic illnesses and other challenges:

https://crohnsandcolitis.org.uk – Crohn's & Colitis UK

https://www.headway.org.uk – *Headway* is the *UK*-wide charity that works to improve life after brain injury by providing vital support and information services.

www.disabledpersons-railcard.co.uk – disabled person's railcard.

Passenger Assist is a service available for older and disabled passengers travelling on the rail network. You contact the network where you are starting the journey to arrange this. Or check out the National Rail enquiries assisted travel pages.

www.tourismforall.co.uk – Tourism for All offers directories of accommodation, things to do, and food and drink to help with planning an accessible holiday.

www.diabetes.co.uk – Diabetes UK, and "DiabetesUK – Know Diabetes. Fight Diabetes", have lots of very useful information on their website, including personal stories of people living with diabetes, eating with diabetes, possible complications, travelling with diabetes, about storing insulin and about glucose monitors.

www.autism.org.uk

Holidays – guide for parents and carers.

www.youngminds.org.uk – also has information on ADHD and travelling with children.

https://adhdinchildrensupport.com/travelling-with-children-with-adhd

About the Author

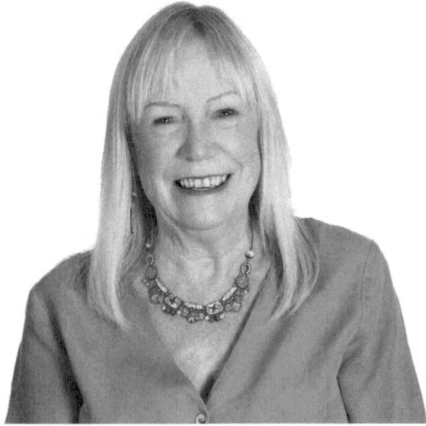

Joanna's love of books started when she was a child, and she read prolifically. This led to studying English in Reading and eventually becoming an English teacher. As part of this journey, Joanna also attended Eastern Michigan University, where she studied American Literature, leading to a fascination with F. Scott Fitzgerald and a subsequent dissertation about his novels. She also studied for a year at the University of Oxford, looking into the area of sex stereotyping in children's fiction and produced a dissertation and various publications focussing on this issue.

Joanna taught English in a school in South Oxfordshire for ten years and she is still in touch with some of her past students, having organised two reunions in recent years. Joanna then moved on to a long career working in different capacities with children with special educational needs and in particular those students with challenging behaviour. She strived to engender in these children a love for reading and writing, even with those who were particularly challenged in these areas. She also became a respite foster carer and recently was nominated to attend a garden party at Buckingham Palace in recognition of her work over many years with children and young people.

Joanna's interest in reading has continued throughout the years. She has an eclectic taste in books and there are still bookcases heaving with books in her house. She has two children and three grandchildren and has always enjoyed reading with them. She loves the fact that her daughter and granddaughter share her passion for reading and exchange recommendations about their favourite books.

Joanna has travelled extensively and has kept journals of some of her trips around the world. More recently, she began to write blogs for forCrohn's, a charity she was involved in, now sadly no longer operational. She raised thousands of pounds for the charity to fund research into Crohn's disease, which she has suffered with since her mid-twenties, organising fundraising events and undertaking challenges in different parts of the world. She wrote these blogs with the intention of encouraging and inspiring people with disabilities to believe that it is still possible to travel to remote locations. This was the inspiration for the book *Gutsy Travels: Travelling the World With My Invisible Friend.*

In 2022, Joanna decided to record the experiences of people she had met around the world, which resulted in the publication of her first book, *Lockdown Stories: Reflections on the pandemic from around the world.*

*   Follow Jo on Facebook: Jo O'Donoghue. Author
*   And on Instagram: @joodonoghueauthor
*   Website: https://joannaodonoghue.co.uk/